PRAISE FOR *RESOLVING THE CR̶I̶S̶I̶S̶ THE KEY ROLE OF BUSINESS CONTINUITY PLANNING*

"One of most common things heard in various institutions goes something like: 'You can't run a (church, school, nonprofit, arts center, university) like a business.' The problem is that people don't understand business and consequently do not define the term correctly. A business is any organization that provides a product or service, collects revenue, and has expenses. Obviously, the university qualifies. As both an experienced academic and a skilled business expert, Dr. Hampton understands that the present plight and questionable future of the traditional university is dependent on creating a business model that works in today's environment. This book not only spells out the problems, but also discusses detailed solutions. It is easy to understand, reads well, and is important to the future of higher education."—**Art Pulis, business consultant, Pulis and Associates**

"There is no question that one of the pillars of strength of a thriving society is an active, robust, forward-thinking educational system. Today, our institutions of higher education are facing enormous challenges—economic, social, health-related concerns—that require clear thinking and solid advice. Dr. Hampton provides just that. In an engaging Socratic manner, he shows us how business continuity planning and risk management are the tools that can help higher education institutions thrive, rather than succumb to outdated and narrow-focused thinking. This book is a must-read requirement for educators, administrators, trustees, government officials, and donors."—**Nathan Sambul, entrepreneur, investor, and visiting professor at universities in the United States and Europe**

"Contemporary university education is more reflective of the medieval format of its origins than of today's fast-paced, technologically advanced society. It is no surprise that new graduates are often woefully unprepared for the knowledge, skills, and abilities required to be successful contributors to the modern workforce. Hampton tackles this disconnect by offering business continuity planning to ameliorate the connection between university instruction and workplace practice. His analysis of the problems presented by traditional liberal arts pedagogy and their contribution to risk in the business of higher education highlights the consequences of 'business as usual.' The apparent bottom line, according to Hampton, is that, as long as universities ignore the importance of revising their business models to reflect contemporary business continuity planning, the new graduate, and thus the contemporary workforce, will allow their work to control them, rather than controlling work for themselves. This insightful piece is a 'must read' for those charged with curriculum development and with enterprise risk management at the university level."—**Elizabeth Mitchell Coronado, PhD, senior training specialist for safety basis, Los Alamos National Laboratory**

"This outstanding book illustrates how the reader can obtain critical facts and apply risk management techniques to make logical decisions in higher education. We know that the choice of college today is a great challenge. Graduates are faced with huge student debt that can take a decade or even longer to repay. Proper planning and the right decisions are needed. The author explains strategies from both the student and college perspective. The book focuses on risk management tools that can be applied to make logical decisions. The author's experience and intensive research produced this exceptional book that encourages readers to pursue critical facts before taking action on a choice of college or careers. The book is a must read for parents of future students. Also, it provides useful information for professors and other college decision makers."—**Gary Seneca, MBA, tax preparer**

"For decades, universities, particularly liberal arts institutions, have overwhelmingly focused on academic pursuits while overlooking the business of education. Their business myopia has resulted in a failure to understand their customers and their products. The COVID-19 pandemic has leveled the playing field for higher education and prompted observant institutions to consider their position in the value chain. In *Resolving the Crisis in Higher Education: The Key Role of Business Continuity Planning*, Hampton demonstrates how modern enterprise risk management could be used to strategically reposition universities to compete in an evolving educational market. He posits that business continuity planning can bring not only sustainability but a competitive advantage to those institutions that embrace the new business plan at all stakeholder levels. Pragmatically written as a series of questions, this book answers the question for anyone competing for higher education's savvy consumers."—**William Fawcett, chief executive officer, Haverford Reinsurance**

"Dr. John J. Hampton has continued his book series on risk management in higher education by heralding risks, particularly to private liberal arts colleges. COVID-19 accelerated those institutional risks, as well as posing new ones. A stakeholder approach to enterprise risk management is urged on boards of trustees, college presidents, administrators, and professors to deal with shared risks and rewards, collaborative governance, and the need to reverse negative trends. Liberal arts education is not at all devalued, but rather is recognized as cultivating critical thinking, improving problem solving, and effectively analyzing information. A challenge is issued to reconceptualize curriculum and degrees based on a liberal arts foundation, including under-graduate and graduate degrees in business. Institutions are further encour-aged to develop student-centered and flexible approaches to course offerings, academic calendars, and the cost of college. Dr. Hampton presents a series of invaluable questions and tools to university leadership at all levels to guide the revision and adaptation of an institution's business model and the identi-fication and creation of its value chains."—**Paula Becker Alexander, PhD, JD, associate professor, Seton Hall University, and author of *Corporate Social Responsibility***

Resolving the Crisis in Higher Education

The Key Role of Business Continuity Planning

John "Jack" Hampton

ROWMAN & LITTLEFIELD
Lanham • Boulder • New York • London

Published by Rowman & Littlefield
An imprint of The Rowman & Littlefield Publishing Group, Inc.
4501 Forbes Boulevard, Suite 200, Lanham, Maryland 20706
www.rowman.com

6 Tinworth Street, London SE11 5AL, United Kingdom

British Library Cataloguing in Publication Information Available

Library of Congress Cataloging-in-Publication Data

Names: Hampton, John, 1942– author.
Title: Resolving the crisis in higher education : the key role of business
    continuity planning / John "Jack" Hampton.
Description: Lanham, Maryland : Rowman & Littlefield, 2021. | Includes
    index. | Summary: "Colleges were created because society needed
    clergymen, philosophers, and scientists. They morphed into producing
    better farmers, factory workers, and office administrators. Now, they
    must prepare young people for a changing world of technology and complex
    systems. This book shows how universities change their business models
    to achieve that goal"—Provided by publisher.
Identifiers: LCCN 2021006917 (print) | LCCN 2021006918 (ebook) | ISBN
    9781475861679 (cloth) | ISBN 9781475861686 (paperback) | ISBN
    9781475861693 (epub)
Subjects: LCSH: Universities and colleges—United States—Business
    management. | Education, Higher—Aims and objectives—United States. |
    COVID-19 Pandemic, 2020–
Classification: LCC LB2341.93.U6 H36 2021 (print) | LCC LB2341.93.U6
    (ebook) | DDC 378.1/06—dc23
LC record available at https://lccn.loc.gov/2021006917
LC ebook record available at https://lccn.loc.gov/2021006918

Contents

Figures

Preface

In the midst of a crisis in higher education in the United States, we might ask a question using the old reliable multiple-choice format:

Which of the following is the goal of a college or university?

A. Prepare individuals to be clergymen, doctors, or lawyers
B. Improve agriculture
C. Create factory and office workers
D. Something else

Before we get to the answer, let's address the reality that an attack by an overwhelming force has targeted higher education. On one side are critics who say a college degree is no longer needed. On another side are parents and students who say a college education has become an expensive waste of time and money. We can explicitly recognize that professors and students are caught in the middle.

We know the criticisms.

- A college education does not prepare students for the lives they'll lead and the careers they'll pursue.
- Many colleges and universities are on government and accreditor financial deficiency watch lists.
- Part-time instructors are replacing full-time professors and tenure is disappearing.
- Students are graduating, or failing to graduate, burdened by excessive levels of debt.

- Legislators are turning away from financially supporting four-year college programs.
- Professors are hired and rewarded for research and oftentimes not held accountable for helping students learn.

From this list of accusations, we can further recognize a chorus of voices recommending nontraditional behaviors for colleges and universities. These include the following:

- Taking advantage of the benefits of online teaching
- Adopting flexible course structures and delivery models
- Offering courses that are more relevant and timely
- Expanding opportunities that enhance teamwork and career readiness

Many presidents, deans, and professors see the need for change. They should get in the game, developing or revising a sustainable business model accompanied by a viable value chain.

A problem arises as many colleges and universities fail to understand and communicate how they create and deliver value. Their effort needs to be accompanied by a strategy that allows them to be rewarded for bringing value to their students and beyond.

This statement will bring an immediate protest on many campuses. Wait a minute. Don't they have published descriptions of their mission, vision, and values?

Of course they do:

- Mission statement: Our university educates . . . learners . . . to excel intellectually, lead ethically, serve compassionately . . .
- Vision statement: Our university has a historic opportunity to . . .
- Values statement: We are an academic community committed to high standards . . . excellence . . . preparing students for lives of learning, leadership, and service.

Good stuff all, but that's about it. These statements do not answer urgent questions from potential students:

- How am I, or my family, going to pay for college?
- Why do I have to take so many courses that don't interest me?
- Why do so many courses repeat the same material I learned in high school?
- How do I blend together attending college and holding down a job?

In the following pages, we show how the survival of many colleges and universities will depend on their success with business continuity planning—the process of developing or revising an obsolete business model and value chain. The logic stream answers a series of questions:

- Current business models: Why are so many of them nonexistent or faulty? Why do they need to be supported by a value chain?
- Enterprise risk management (ERM): How does this powerful tool help identify and manage the full spectrum of risks facing higher education?
- Business continuity plan (BCP): How does a university create a BCP task force that will actually develop a sustainable long-term survival strategy?
- Key role of the liberal arts: How does it fit in a sustainable value chain for a university?
- Modern curriculum: How can we build it on a liberal arts foundation?
- Role of key stakeholders: What do we need from professors, administrators, and trustees?

Before starting on our journey, we return to our multiple-choice question.

Question: Which of the following is the goal of a college or university?
Answer:

A. To prepare individuals to be clergymen, doctors, or lawyers? The answer is yes, particularly in the period from 1740 to 1820.
B. To improve agriculture? Yes, starting in about 1820.
C. To create factory and office workers? Yes, starting in about 1870, expanding after 1920, and going crazy with technology since the birth of the internet.
D. Something else? Yes. Today, the best answer recognizes that the primary goal is survival.

Our university works to understand student needs and motivations and match them with programs that deliver the knowledge and skills they need in a financial package that provides sustainable long-term viability for the school.

Colleges and universities that pursue this goal supported by the right value chain increase their chances for long-term survival.

In plain English, the goal of this book is to start the reader on a journey from today to tomorrow through the lens of business continuity planning. It reaffirms the importance of the liberal arts as a foundation for life and work. It identifies business models that offer value and flexibility with a goal to create viable and sustainable activities into a confusing future for higher education. It challenges traditional behaviors to retain the best of what professors and universities do and get rid of all the junk that blocks the road.

Happy journey.

John "Jack" Hampton
Litchfield, Connecticut, November 2020

Chapter One

Do Liberal Arts Colleges Have Viable Business Models? Even More Important, Why Do They Need Them?

THE LIBERAL ARTS

The liberal arts originated in ancient Greece as the knowledge and skills needed to take an active part in citizenship. In medieval universities, it comprised seven areas obscurely known as the trivium and quadrivium. The three lower-level subjects were grammar, rhetoric, and logic and the four upper division areas were arithmetic, music, geometry, and astronomy.

Today, liberal arts refers to a collection of academic subjects in two distinct categories:

- General education: A liberal arts foundation refers to courses that instill a common cultural heritage during the first two years of full-time undergraduate studies.
- Liberal arts education: A liberal arts degree or field of study refers to in-depth study in one of the areas covered in the courses that form the cultural heritage. Examples are English, history, philosophy, economics, and psychology.

LIBERAL ARTS FOUNDATION

With respect to the liberal arts as general education, most observers of higher education value the liberal arts foundation. They have widespread agreement on the value of the expected learning outcomes. These can be grouped into two categories:

- Intellectual and practical skills: Inquiry, analysis, critical and creative thinking, written and oral communication, reading, information literacy, and problem solving
- Personal and social responsibility: Local and global civic engagement, intercultural knowledge and competence, ethical reasoning, and skills for lifelong and global learning

DISAGREEMENT ON ACHIEVING THE OUTCOMES

If most observers respect the liberal arts, fierce disagreement can arise in the details of program design. Stakeholders in the university often hold strong divergent beliefs about aspects of the academic model. Figure 1.1 identifies issues to be resolved in the liberal arts foundation.

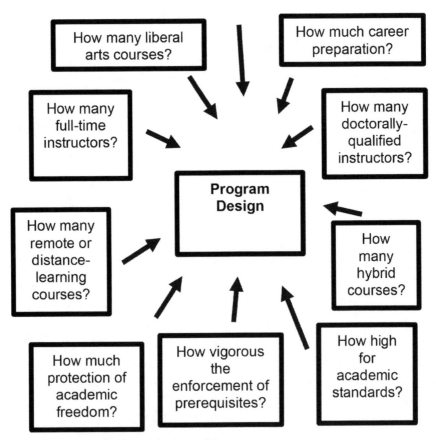

Figure 1.1.   Issues in the Academic Model

Traditionally, battle lines have been drawn between professors, administrators, students, parents, and alumni as to the content of the liberal arts foundation. Issues include the following:

- How much liberal arts is needed? Schools have different views of the number of courses to be required in a core curriculum that comprise the liberal arts foundation. The length varies from school to school, ranging between 30 and 66 credits in a 120-credit-hour undergraduate degree program.
- Who should make academic decisions? Random discussions are often introduced to justify different points of view. Conflict arises among faculty, administrators, trustees, and students. Liberal arts programs in colleges are often contrasted with other areas of study that are primarily vocational, professional, or technical. Therein lies the rub. Many voices are growing louder on the role of the liberal arts.
- How relevant are the liberal arts anyway? This core of a college degree is a cultural heritage of the medieval beginning of modern higher education. Professors agree on the concept of general education but disagree on what it should include. Requirements essentially evolve in silos where departments battle to get their courses included. Outside forces and sponsors weigh in. A college supported by a religious body might have two philosophy and two theology courses. A secular institution might have social responsibility and community service.
- Bachelor of science versus bachelor of arts: A lingering issue in the academy deals with the differences between a BA and BS degree. A bachelor of arts is a broad interdisciplinary program of general education. A bachelor of science is more specialized. This distinction does not stand up well to scrutiny. For a degree such as economics, a university may award a BS or a BA degree.
- Liberal arts college: A liberal arts institution requires a general education core containing the humanities, arts, sciences, and social sciences. When this is completed, students may choose a major in the liberal arts or other fields such as business or education.

COMPARING A LIBERAL ARTS LECTURE
AND A TYPEWRITER

Before getting into a discussion on the value of a traditional college education, we might answer a simple question.

Question: Does a modern university built around professorial lectures resemble a company that makes typewriters?

Answer: Perhaps in one way. We can describe a resemblance between the lecture format and, for example, a Smith Corona or Royal Typewriter.

Essentially, there is nothing wrong with a manual or even electric typewriter. You can still buy one today on Amazon or at Staples. It is more difficult to find out who makes them. Consider two memorable brand names:

- Smith Corona: This company made its first typewriter in 1886 and its last in 2013. Although it stopped making typewriters many years ago, its online typewriter museum is open twenty-four hours a day, year-round, at https://www.smithcorona.com/blog/gallery/.
- Royal Typewriter: Known by a different name today, the company manufactures electronic office supplies, weather stations, imaging supplies, and more. It does not sell typewriters.

The comparison with today's universities arises because many college classrooms share the fate of the typewriter. Nothing wrong with them other than technology has made them inefficient.

- You can still type a paper with a typewriter. Why would you bother when a personal computer allows much easier corrections, revisions, and sharing of a document?
- You can still take notes in a college lecture hall. Why would you bother when technology allows you to learn more at your own pace in an often interactive and even entertaining format?

MISSION, VISION, AND VALUES STATEMENTS

Today, the comparison with the typewriter is in the forefront of rising demands for reforms in U.S. higher education. Just like people did with typewriters, many parents and students are asking such questions as

- Does everyone need college education?
- If yes, what kind of learning should take place?

Universities have never ignored these questions. They distribute their answers in recruiting brochures, academic catalogues, and website postings. They emphatically proclaim their response to these challenges in three forms—mission, vision, and values statements. Expanding on the statements in the preface, we get the following:

Mission statement: Defines the school's goals and activity to achieve them. Example: Our university, inspired by its Christian identity, commitment to individual attention, and grounding in the liberal arts, educates a diverse community of learners in undergraduate, graduate, and professional programs to excel intellectually, lead ethically, serve compassionately, and promote justice in our ever-changing economic and global environment.

Vision statement: Describes the desired future position of the school. Example: Our university has a historic opportunity to build on its traditions and strengths while deepening its commitment to providing an outstanding liberal arts education. Four initiatives—strengthen long-term finances, increase voluntary giving, further communication strategies, and assess progress—will support organizational effectiveness and help to secure our future.

Values statement: Paints a picture of how the university sees itself. Example: We are an academic community committed to high standards and the pursuit of excellence. The community is built on a partnership between students who accept responsibility as fully engaged learners and the university dedicated to offering quality instruction and excellent services. Students can expect a vibrant learning environment characterized by individual respect and ethical values. All activities prepare students for lives of learning, leadership, and service.

Question: Is there a problem with these mission, vision, and values statements?

Answer: Yes. Universities often do not accompany the statements with a plan to pursue their goals. Instead, they stop after praising how good it is to be us. Consider the following:

- Mission statement: "Our university, inspired by its . . ."
- Vision statement: "Our university has a historic opportunity to build on its traditions and strengths . . ."
- Values statement: We are an academic community . . . high standards . . . pursuit of excellence . . ."

Thus, we have a problem. To augment its mission and other statements, many universities need more robust strategic planning. They should address risk and opportunity every time they examine their priorities and recognize the need to make changes.

KEY TERMS

Before tackling strategic planning in higher education, we need to define a few terms:

- Business model: A statement that shows how an organization creates and delivers value and is rewarded for bringing it to others
- Value chain: A set of activities that an organization performs to deliver a valuable product or service to a market
- Value chain analysis: A process to determine which activities are the most valuable and which need to be improved
- Long-term sustainable viability: A situation where an organization has a business model and value chain that is likely to support growth and/or survival into the distant future

A business model is built upon a value chain analysis that identifies risks and expected benefits. It can apply to individual degrees, schools, disciplines, or the entire university. It seeks to provide the pathway to long-term sustainable viability.

A SIMPLE BUSINESS MODEL AND VALUE CHAIN

To illustrate building a business model, consider a college student who is evaluating selling hot dogs at the beach during a ten-week summer break. The student will purchase hot dogs, buns, mustard, and other supplies from a wholesaler, obtain a license from the city, rent two hot dog wagons, and hire a classmate to help sell at two different locations. The student estimates selling price, costs, the level of sales, and the likely number of sunny days and puts all the information in a value chain. Table 1.1 shows that expected profit is a measure of the viability of the venture.

Looking good. But what happens if he faces competition and has to lower the selling price? Table 1.2 shows the impact. Still good, but nowhere close to the original profit number.

Finally, what about the viability if multiple inputs turn out to be inaccurate? Table 1.3 shows the impact of a lower selling price, fewer hot dogs sold daily, and fewer sunny beach days.

Question: What does the value chain analysis tell us about the viability of the hot dog wagon project?

Answer: If the initial inputs are based on logic, accurate cost data, and other evidence, the analysis shows a viable business model with a limited

Table 1.1. Value Chain Analysis

	Inputs	Cash Flow
Selling price, hot dog, etc.	$5	
Hot dogs sold daily	200	
Forecast of sunny days	60	
Summer revenues		$60,000
#1 Cart rental, summer	$600	
#2 Cart rental, summer	$600	
License fee	$300	
Startup costs		−$1,500
Cost of hot dogs	$1	
Hot dogs sold daily	200	
Forecast of sunny days	60	
Hot dogs, total cost		−$12,000
Hourly cost, self	$0	
Hourly cost, classmate	$15	
Total hourly cost	$15	
Hours worked daily	8	
Forecast of sunny days	60	
Workers, total costs		−$7,200
Expected profit/loss		$39,300

Table 1.2. Sensitivity of the Selling Price Assumption

	Inputs	Cash Flow
Selling price, hot dog, etc.	$3	
Hot dogs sold daily	200	
Forecast of sunny days	60	
Summer revenues		$36,000
#1 Cart rental, summer	$600	
#2 Cart rental, summer	$600	
License fee	$300	
Startup costs		−$1,500
Cost of hot dogs	$1	
Hot dogs sold daily	200	
Forecast of sunny days	60	
Hot dogs, total cost		−$12,000
Hourly cost, self	$0	
Hourly cost, classmate	$15	
Total hourly cost	$15	
Hours worked daily	8	
Forecast of sunny days	60	
Workers, total costs		−$7,200
Expected profit/loss		$15,300

downside risk. Yes, the student could actually lose a little money, but three of the inputs would have to prove to be inaccurate for this to happen.

Table 1.3. Sensitivity of Assumptions, Selling Price, Daily Sales, and Number of Sunny Days

	Inputs	Cash Flow
Selling price, hot dog, etc.	$2	
Hot dogs sold daily	120	
Forecast of sunny days	50	
Summer revenues		$12,000
#1 Cart rental, summer	$600	
#2 Cart rental, summer	$600	
License fee	$300	
Startup costs		-$1,500
Cost of hot dogs	$1	
Hot dogs sold daily	120	
Forecast of sunny days	50	
Hot dogs, total cost		-$6,000
Hourly cost, self	$0	
Hourly cost, classmate	$15	
Total hourly cost	$15	
Hours worked daily	8	
Forecast of sunny days	50	
Workers, total costs		-$6,000
Expected profit/loss		-$1,500

BUSINESS MODEL FOR A UNIVERSITY

Giving best wishes to the college student for a successful summer project, we move on to examples of academic business models:

- Our university works to understand student needs and motivations and match them with programs that deliver knowledge they need and want in a financial package that provides sustainable long-term viability of the school.

This is a slightly different model:

- We offer degrees and courses to traditional-age students while recognizing different socio and economic backgrounds and matching different needs and goals in multiple programs designed to create a financially sustainable business model.

Next, we discuss backing up the business model with a value chain that connects academic products and student services with parents and students. In this process, we ask a series of questions:

- Value of academic product or service: What do parents and students want or need from the university?
- Identification of a specific market: Who should pay for college and why would they want to pay?
- Resources, including partnerships, to create and deliver knowledge: What are our capabilities to meet myriad student needs even as we try to educate them in various forums and methodology?
- Delivery activities and channel(s): Do we have a vibrant and flexible approach to delivering academic products? If not, how can we successfully compete in an overcrowded market that inevitably and significantly will decline in the near future?
- Cash inflow and outflow projections during the span of a planning period: What are the prospects for our current efforts and proposed reforms? What does the business model do to enhance the likelihood of our long-term sustainable viability?

VALUE CHAIN FOR A CALLIGRAPHY DEGREE

We can now apply the value chain analysis to a proposal for a new degree in calligraphy.

Question: A donor has offered a university $5 million to establish an undergraduate calligraphy degree program. The proposal seeks to reverse the decline of skills in the art of Latin, Greek, and Cyrillic writing and penmanship as practiced in the Western world. Should the institution establish and offer the program?

Answer: Maybe. One way to answer the question is to complete a value chain analysis.

- Value of a calligraphy degree: A quick check of U.S. college courses identified no degree program in calligraphy (https://www.postgrad.com /courses/calligraphy/usa/any-attendance/masters/). The subject is covered in some fine arts programs. If demand exists for such a degree, the United States presently has no competition.
- Identification of a target market: Who wants to be a calligrapher? A career explorer website provides information on the profession (https://www .careerexplorer.com/careers/calligrapher/job-market/):

- There are thirteen thousand active calligraphers working in the United States, with a concentration in Washington, DC, and California.
- The majority of students interested in calligraphy as a career choice earn a degree in fine arts, since calligraphy can be associated with design, graphics, and typography.
- The website gives the field an F employability rating, meaning this career is expected to provide poor employment opportunities for the foreseeable future.
- Resources, including partnerships, to create and deliver knowledge:
  - The $5 million endowment will allow the university to provide scholarships. To some degree, this frees the school from a dependency on tuition.
  - The university may be able to work with the International Association of Master Penmen, Engrossers and Teachers of Handwriting (IAMPETH), an association of one thousand members who practice and preserve the arts of calligraphy.
  - IAMPETH may also be a competitor as it offers certificates of proficiency, excellence, and master penmanship.
- Delivery activities and channel(s): It is not clear that a university—any university—has devised channels to reach potential applicants for a calligraphy program. Many have fine arts programs with occasional calligraphy courses.
- Cash inflow and outflow projections during the span of a planning period: This is a complete unknown even within the framework of a $5 million endowment.

Question: After reading the report on the value chain analysis for a calligraphy degree, the university president asks the dean, "What is your best-case, expectation, and worst-case estimate of the number of students in the program?" What is a valid answer?

Answer: We're hoping for twenty students. We expect fewer. We may get none at all.

The dean's answer does not reflect a refusal to develop new programs. Instead, it deals with the reality that a calligraphy degree is supported by a weak value chain. Instead of offering the degree, the institution may try to direct the donor to the fine arts, where calligraphy could be a component of the degree.

If every program were subject to a value chain analysis, many programs offered today would be dropped by their universities. Perhaps this explains the somewhat quirky faculty and administrator views on business models and value chains.

FACULTY VIEW OF A VALUE CHAIN

Whether in the *Chronicle of Higher Education*, the faculty lounge, or the classroom, professors are not shy about discussing their views on current conditions on the campus. Many of their ideas do not align with a viable business model. If you take the time to locate the grumpiest member of the faculty, you can learn a dark view of a value chain:

- Value of the degree: It is our job to teach in our relatively narrow of area of expertise. We're mostly not curious about student goals after graduation. We tell them what we know, which may have little connection to their goals, and then carry on with our research or largely mindless and meaningless tasks that are part of the duties of a professor.
- Need of a specific market: We don't know where the recruiters find some of these students. We want the admissions office to bring us students who are smart enough to agree with our views.
- Resources: This is not our concern. Colleges should not be run like businesses in any case.
- Delivery activities and channel(s): The administration should figure this out without affecting what we do with our students.
- Cash inflow and outflow projections during the span of a planning period: Not our concern. We already told you. Colleges and universities are not businesses.

ADMINISTRATOR VIEW OF A VALUE CHAIN

A second explanation for the lack of support for value chain analysis can be found in the university administration. The president, dean, admissions officers, and other administrators are often trained by people who do not know how to create and deliver value for others. Rather, they are familiar with academic and administrative processes that deliver, in many cases, little value. You might find an unhappy administrator who describes a value chain like this:

- Value of the degree: It is not our business. Professors control the programs, curriculums, and courses.
- Need of a specific market: We want the admissions office to bring us students. That's about it.
- Resources: It's our concern but there is little we can do about resources without faculty cooperation, which is unlikely. Plus, everybody is fighting

for a piece of a continually declining pot of money. What can we do but seek our share whether we need it or not?

- Delivery activities and channel(s): If we have to do something, let's copy the efforts of others. Maybe they know what to do.
- Cash inflow and outflow projections during the span of a planning period: Maybe some of the copied activities will bring in money.

CONCLUSION

We can't be too critical of the value of a university's idealized mission, vision, and values statements. Its stakeholders want to think of themselves as belonging to a community where professors and administrators are doing a good job even as they aspire to be better. Even so, the future of many colleges and universities in the United States is in jeopardy if they do not prepare to respond to changing conditions in higher education. To do this, many need a new business model and value chain.

Chapter Two

What Is the Risk of a Faulty Business Model? Do Professors and Administrators Need to Work Together to Get It Right?

STRATEGY AND TACTICS

The creation of a business model is the responsibility of top management: the president and senior executives of a university. The trustees should ensure that the process distinguishes between strategies and tactics, as follows:

- Strategy: This is an approach to achieving a goal selected after a review of various alternatives. During the planning process, declining a strategic goal is possible.
- Tactic: This is an approach to achieving a goal when declining the goal is not possible.

Question: The board of trustees directed the president to examine the viability of an emergency medical services (EMS) bachelor's degree. Is this a request to pursue a strategic or tactical goal?
Answer: Without further information, it appears to be strategic. The president can advise the board of the findings and the board can evaluate it on its merits.

Question: The president asked the academic vice president to prepare an application for a $3 million grant from the National Highway Traffic Safety Administration to offer an EMS bachelor's degree. Is this a request to pursue a strategic or tactical goal?
Answer: It looks like a tactical goal. The academic vice president may not have the choice to decline to draft the recommendation.

STRATEGIC PURPOSE

Peter Drucker claims that the only strategic goal of an organization is to create a customer. Such a goal statement orients a university to ensure its business model answers specific questions:

- What is the value of our degrees and student experiences?
- Who are our students?
- Why are they enrolling in our courses?

Although important, these questions do not provide all the information needed to support the business model.

Question: A school has been training secretarial assistants to executives for many years. The school graduates individuals with excellent shorthand notation and typing skills. Even so, enrollments were rapidly declining. The school evaluated its value chain. What did it find out?
Answer: It learned:

- Current degrees? Students learn how to type and take shorthand.
- Current students? Students are future office workers.
- Motives to enroll? Students intend to get jobs as secretaries and administrative assistants.

These answers are accurate but reflect skills that are declining in importance as career fields.

Question: What should the school ask about its value chain?
Answer:

- What will be the value of our degrees and student experience?
- Who will be our students?
- How do we create new programs with students in new value chains that have sustainable viability?

The strategic purpose of a university is to prepare students for the future. When academic programs are not aligned with a changing business model, adjustments need to be made.

- Degrees: Are they the right topics?
- Students: Are we aligned with the needs of our target students?
- Value chain: Is it still viable?

COMPONENTS OF A VALUE CHAIN

It's an easy transition to move from a generalized business model to a value chain that fits the typical college or university. The components are

- Value of an academic experience: Our degrees are credentials that are worth the cost and effort to achieve them.
- Need of a specific market: Programs are designed to be attractive to a target cohort with similar goals, backgrounds, or needs.
- Resources: The institution provides adequate resources to deliver programs that will meet the value desired by, and at a price suitable to, the target market.
- Delivery activities and channel(s): Programs are supported by a stable and efficient supply chain that contains recruiting, admissions, enrollment, course offerings, and support services.
- Cash inflow and outflow projections during the span of a planning period: Activities are designed and monitored so they produce an adequate return for the risk in our investment.

Figure 2.1 shows these components.

DESIGN THINKING IS RECOMMENDED

After identifying the components, we need a process to engage the right people in value chain analysis. Design thinking is a popular format to consider when building or revising a business model and its value chain.

- It starts by identifying and using knowledge to develop strategic and practical processes and behaviors.
- It encourages group participation and visual referencing tools to gather information.
- It pursues an evaluation of the opportunities that are expected from the business model.
- It delineates the risks that may undermine or destroy the goals of the model.

For a university, the strategic planning technique identifies a team that examines the capabilities of the institution and the needs of potential students. Then, the team uses its knowledge to design and offer attractive degree or other programs.

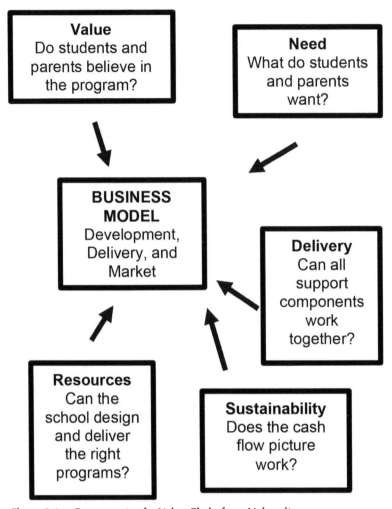

Figure 2.1. Components of a Value Chain for a University

Design thinking seeks innovative solutions to often complex problems. It arose in response to an emerging reality for many areas of activity, including higher education. Stated simply: Since society is constantly moving and everything is changing, change is not an exception. Rather, change is the norm.

ISSUES WHEN DEVELOPING A VALUE CHAIN

The process of developing a value chain takes place in a risk management and strategic planning context that includes both foreseeable risk and benefits of opportunity. Some issues in the balancing act include the following:

- Wicked problems: These are ill defined or tricky, as opposed to wicked in the sense of malicious. Academia seems to prefer well-defined problems where a solution is available through applying rules or technical knowledge.
- Problem framing: This is process of refusing to accept the problem as initially stated. The organization explores the issues and reinterprets or restructures the problem in a way that suggests options to make needed changes.
- Solution-focused thinking: This is a behavior to find a solution to move forward rather than identify the causes of a problem. When people seek to solve a problem, a narrow focus often wastes time while failing to pursue innovative remedies to manage change.
- Abductive reasoning: This refers to the search for a simple and most likely solution to a problem. The team does not try to find the "perfect" solution. Rather, it often agrees to a workable or likely to succeed solution and approves it.
- Circular rotation of problem and solution: Design thinking starts with problem statements and tries to identify solutions, revise statements and refine solutions, and repeat the process, triggering innovative solutions.
- Visual modeling: The innovation team using design thinking tries to communicate mostly using visual models or representations of problems, actions, and solutions.

Figure 2.2 shows a visual model of these risk management issues.

THREE DETERMINANTS OF VALUE

From the context of risk and opportunity, design thinking pursues the challenge for higher education. This requires moving away from past assumptions and viewpoints to a viewpoint of the activities that create value. A university is a composite of three separate determinants of value:

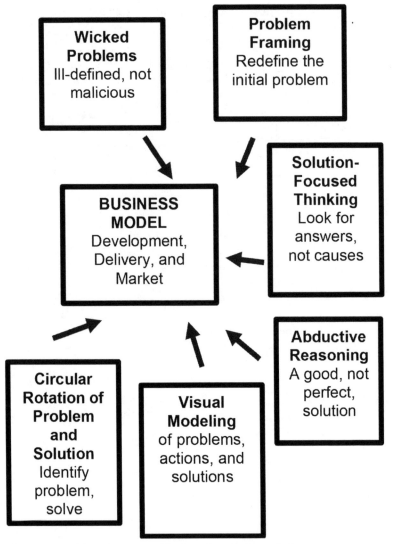

Figure 2.2.   **Risk and Opportunities in Value Chain Analysis**

- Academic innovation: Essentially, this involves degree, certificate, career preparation, continuing education, and other programs targeted to specific audiences. It includes curriculum and course design.
- Relationship management: Dealing with students, alumni, external communities, government agencies, and others in various capacities.

- Infrastructure management: Creating an institutional structure that supports all activities and delivers according to required standards.

Figure 2.3 shows the determinants of value using design thinking.

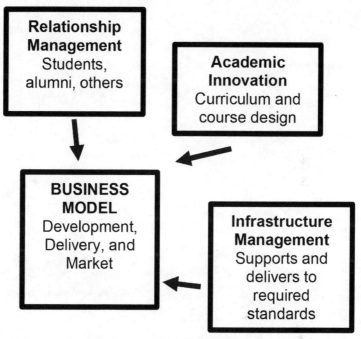

Figure 2.3.   Determinants of Value in a Business Model

RISK FACTORS IN VALUE CHAINS

A university has a risk management task dealing with three aspects of each of the business model activities:

- Economics: Operating within fixed parameters that allow a program to achieve specific financial goals
- Competition: Developing strategies to be successful in a competitive marketplace
- Culture: Creating a culture that fits the value system and attracts qualified individuals to work together to achieve goals

Figure 2.4 addresses the risks to include in the discussion.

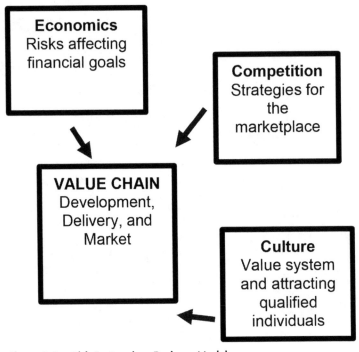

Figure 2.4.   Risk Factors in a Business Model

MARKET INSIGHTS IN VALUE CHAINS

A market insight is an interpretation of a behavior or situation that explains the needs and likely behavior of individuals in a target market. When an insight **is** accurately a penetrating truth, activities can be designed to meet needs and achieve success.

A value chain for most universities requires a specific focus on tuition revenues. An innovation team can identify and evaluate specific actions:

- Increase the cost per credit hour by 20 percent to increase total tuition by 20 percent
- Decrease the cost per credit hour by 20 percent to attract more students
- Offer new degree programs
- Lower admissions standards

- Raise admissions standards
- Advertise on television
- Advertise on billboards
- Advertise on Instagram or Snapchat

Question: Which one of the options to raise tuition works best?
Answer: None of these. All off them are fraught with risk and uncertainty. The only way to make a choice is to develop a business model for each option.

Figure 2.5 shows the areas that need their own design thinking models in the development of a business strategy.

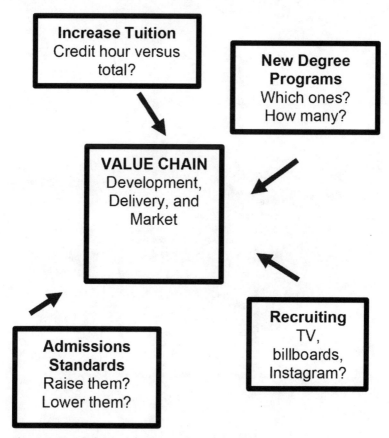

Figure 2.5. Market Insights in a Value Chain

STRATEGIES OF A BUSINESS MODEL

Figure 2.6 shows a university business model based on two quite different strategies.

- Organization-centric strategy: We examine our products, capabilities, skills, and resources. We figure out an academic or nonacademic program and offer it. We estimate the size of different markets. We price the product to make money, offer it to consumers, and hope for the best.
- Customer-centric strategy: We identify the needs of potential students and their families. We figure out a way to help them at a price they are willing to pay. We develop a product that meets their needs. We price the product to make money, offer. . . . You know the rest.

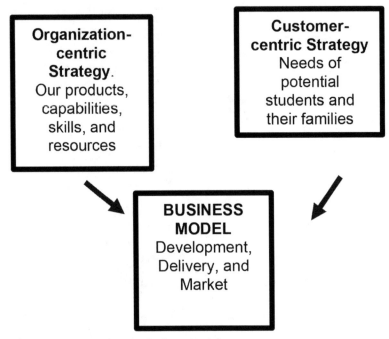

Figure 2.6.   Strategies of a Business Model

The difference between an organization-centric and a customer-centric strategy is whether we talk or listen.

Question: "This is what we have and are offering to sell." What kind of strategy is this? Does it involve talking or listening?
Answer: Organization-centric. It is a talking strategy.

Question: What is the question matching the customer-based strategy?
Answer: "What is it that we need to develop to meet your needs?" It is a listening strategy.

CUSTOMER-BASED BUSINESS MODEL

Colleges and universities need to learn how to use a customer-based strategy to build a business model. Figure 2.7 shows its characteristics. Aspects include the following:

- Perception: What do others see when they look at us? Do they see a valuable potential partner, a friend, or an entity that might have something useful to improve their lives?
- Influence: What do others hear about us from their friends, bosses, teachers, neighbors, family, and other influencers? Are they saying good things, bad things, nothing?
- Behaviors: How do others perceive our activities and our value? Is it good, bad, indifferent, or nonexistent?
- Beliefs: What do others think and feel about their lives, fortunes, abilities, strengths, and weaknesses? How do we know what they believe? Can we tailor messages to deal with misinformation and bias that shapes opinions, assumptions, and feelings?
- Pain: What does not work with potential consumers? What are their concerns and fears? What are the frustrations and obstacles that cause them to struggle?
- Joy: What do they want or need to improve their lives? How do they measure achievement? What is their idea of success?

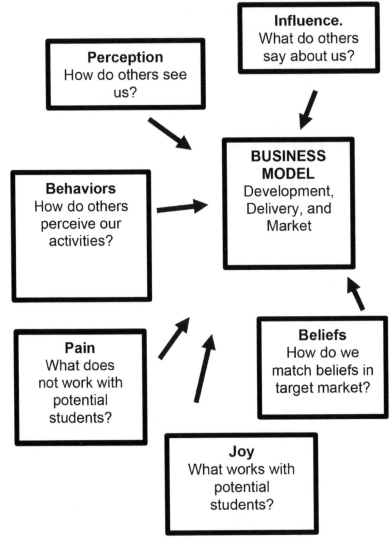

Figure 2.7.   Components of Customer-Based Strategy to Developing a Business Model

CONCLUSION

A university needs to pay attention to the nature of a business model and the issues that arise in value chain analysis to succeed. Design thinking can help create the context for effectively creating a value chain for sustainable long-term viability.

Chapter Three

Does Your University Know about Enterprise Risk Management? Or Will Risks Simply Take Care of Themselves?

ENTERPRISE RISK MANAGEMENT

It is one thing to recognize that colleges and universities face the same array of risks as other organizations. It is quite another to address risks properly in business models and value chains. Let's take a look.

Enterprise risk is the variability of risks and opportunities when organizations conduct their operations. It is a double-edged sword, as it focuses on an upside and a downside.

- Missed opportunity: The failure to undertake a risk when it provides economic value possibilities at an acceptable level of risk
- Financial loss: The exposures that arise from a university's activities that can cause losses to current economic value

Question: A university is evaluating a new bachelor of science degree program. The projection is that the school will enroll one hundred students and graduate twenty-two of them annually once the program is fully operational. At the projected enrollment level, the program will generate an annual $400,000 of tuition exceeding expenses. If enrollments drop below fifty students, the program will have a $100,000 annual negative cash flow. What kind of enterprise risk is involved?
Answer: Both kinds. If it does not achieve fifty students, it will have a financial loss. If it decides not to approve the program, it misses the opportunity to have a positive cash flow.

Enterprise risk management is the process of managing losses and seizing opportunities as the two sides of managing risk in organizations. Related to the achievement of a school's objectives. ERM encourages colleges and universities to perform certain tasks:

- Identify courses of action, developments, circumstances, and behaviors
- Assess them in terms of likelihood and severity of negative impact or lost opportunity
- Develop a strategy to reduce risk or seize opportunity
- Monitor the progress toward objectives

The ERM process is designed to protect students, professors, employees, and others from harm and create value for all stakeholders and supporters of an institution.

BUSINESS RISK

ERM tells us it is a new world of risk for higher education. No longer is risk management largely limited to the isolated silos of classrooms, athletics, recruiting, housing and feeding, or other activities that define college life. We do not assume that the admissions office is responsible for enrollments any more than the bursar is accountable for shortfalls in cash flow.

The institutional risk picture is incomplete when limited to the individual academic or administrative components of a university. This realization encourages new approaches to bringing together trustees, professors, administrators, students, and alumni to balance an institution's appetite for risk, avoid unacceptable exposures, and make changes when needed for prosperity or survival.

Business risk refers to the exposure that an organization will fail to meet its target or achieve its financial goals. For a university, this includes

- Risk associated with the unique circumstances of changes in a marketplace for educational services in a variety of settings
- A situation, either the result of internal conditions or external factors, that may have a negative impact on enrollments, alumni donations, or other financial support
- The possibility of a destructive shift in the circumstances, assumptions, or beliefs that are used in planning and delivering programs and services to achieve educational and financial goals

Sometimes the benefit from a taking course of action is accompanied by an offsetting loss from not making a change. As an example, a school might be discussing outsourcing a campus bookstore to a third party. The proponents discuss efficiency. The opponents point out lost services that are a likely part of the agreement. ERM takes a look at the total picture before making a decision.

ADDRESSING BUSINESS RISK

Organizations have two ways to address risk. The wrong way is to assume that people can understand hundreds or even thousands of exposures. It is not possible. Risks and opportunities must be organized and accepted at various levels by risk owners. Figure 3.1 contains a brief overview of ERM that includes the following specific features:

- Upside of risk: Most people discuss risk as the possibility of loss. This is totally insufficient, as risk also has an upside. A lost opportunity is just as much a financial loss as damage to people and property. This is a key insight. Ask the ancient Chinese warrior Sun-Tzu or the fictional *Godfather* character Michael Corleone.
- Alignment with the business model: Within its business model, a university has a hierarchy where a vice president supervises deans who supervise departments, professors, students, and staff. Each risk manager oversees

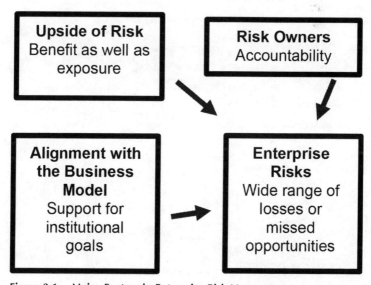

Figure 3.1. Major Factors in Enterprise Risk Management

a limited number of risks and initiatives. ERM encourages us to align the hierarchy of risk categories with the business model.

- Risk owners: Just as someone is accountable for revenues, profits, and efficiency in each organizational unit, a single person should be responsible for every category of risk. When questions arise, we are not dealing with a committee or multiple individuals. We go directly to the risk owner. Even as we say this, some risk assessments must be shared. Exposures in the culture, leadership, or even reputation of the institution should be assessed using collaboration among administrators, professors, and others.

QUESTIONS ABOUT ERM

Like so many concepts in the management of a university, the term enterprise risk management raises various issues. Figure 3.2 poses questions:

- Is it limited to financial risks such as excessive debt or a shortage of cash?
- Does it cover operational risk of business interruption, economic downturns, or natural disasters?

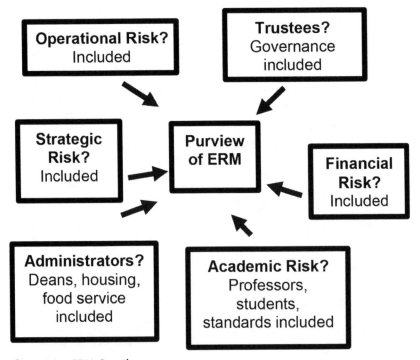

Figure 3.2. ERM Questions

- How does it differ from strategic risk where the school tries to figure out how to achieve its vision and values?
- Is risk management the sole purview of the trustees and president?
- Are vice presidents, deans, department chairs, and professors exempt from the discussion?

Enterprise risk management takes advantage of many of the marketing, finance, and decision-making tools used by businesses, membership associations, and public and private entities. Effectively, a university must include strategies for creating economic value as part of its planning process. They assist in decision making as the institution assesses risk and seizes opportunity.

This approach to enterprise risk is fundamentally different from earlier definitions. ERM recognizes that every management decision has an upside and downside. Thus, risks are viewed in the realm of uncertainty that can have favorable or unfavorable outcomes. Within this framework, managers identify a variety of exposures and opportunities under the umbrella of risk management.

CATEGORIZING RISK

Enterprise risk management encourages the organizing of risks and opportunities into a hierarchy that matches the business model of an organization. Figure 3.3 shows one structure that creates the following categories:

- Academic and nonacademic activities: Degrees, research projects, programs of study, courses, extracurricular activities, community partnerships, and more
- Recruiting: Efforts to reach students, parents, alumni, donors, research and other funding sources, partners, and more
- Cash flows: Management of cash flows from tuition, academic support, ancillary activities, alumni and other benefactors, government agencies, and others sufficient to fund operations
- Compliance: Aligning activities with legal, regulatory, and accreditation requirements, processes, and guidelines
- Technology: Dealing with changes in systems that support education and research and provide modern information and communications
- Business disruption: Preparing for negative events that slow or cease operations and taking steps to return to normal activity

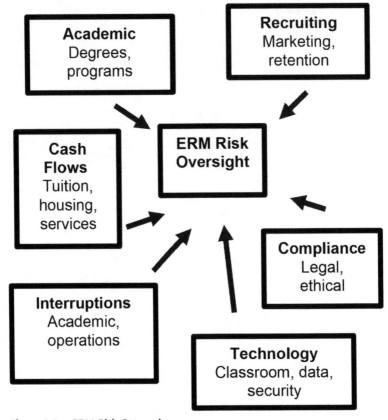

Figure 3.3. ERM Risk Categories

CONCLUSION

Enterprise risk management brings together the perspectives of administrators, professors, and students into a single picture for mitigating negative consequences of decisions and enhancing successful pursuit of new opportunities to allow a modern university to survive and even prosper.

Chapter Four

Why Is Managing the Business Model Similar to Climbing Mount Everest? Are We Sure We Know What We're Doing as We Face Risk in the Immediate Future?

WOULD YOU CONSIDER CLIMBING MOUNT EVEREST?

Within the scope of enterprise risk management, a university should understand the nature of risk in the decision-making process. Let's look at a challenge that has the potential for negative loss or great opportunity.

Question: Can you name an exposure, peril, and hazard associated with climbing Mount Everest?
Answer: Sure.

- Exposure: Agreeing to start climbing is to accept an exposure.
- Perils: We have many choices, including snow blindness, freezing conditions, death, hypothermia, hypoxia, weight loss, severe injury, high-altitude cerebral edema (HACE), and high-altitude pulmonary edema (HAPE).
- Hazards: The climber can increase the already sizeable danger. The chance of death increases when a climber does not carry oxygen or does not train in advance.

Question: How about a successful outcome? Do a lot of people succeed at reaching the top of Mount Everest?
Answer:

- First person to reach the top: Sir Edmund Hillary (1953)
- Successes between 1953–1996: 615
- Successes between 1953–2020: 4,500

31

Question: Do many people die on the mountain?
Answer: Table 4.1 shows that almost three hundred people have died since 1953. This is 6.5 percent of the number who reached the top and returned. Tens of thousands attempted the climb.

**Table 4.1.   Causes of Death
on Mount Everest, 1953–2019**

Cause of Death	Number
Avalanche	68
Fall	67
Exposure	27
Altitude sickness	36
Cardiac/stroke	13
Other or unknown	81
Total	292

SHOULD A UNIVERSITY ACCEPT THE RISKS OF CHANGING ITS BUSINESS MODEL?

Changing the business model contains both risk and opportunity in the ERM framework.

Question: Can you name an exposure, peril, and hazard associated with changing a business model?
Answer: Sure.

- Exposure: Deciding to change it. The journey begins.
- Perils: Key stakeholders may not agree with the need for change or they may have a variety of ideas of the changes that are needed.
- Hazards: The proposed changes can decrease existing behaviors that stabilize the financial, enrollment, or other situations. Closing the wrong programs or allocating funds to new programs carry the danger of miscalculation or denial of resources to currently successful activities.

Question: How about a successful outcome? Do a lot of colleges and universities succeed in their efforts to reinvent themselves?
Answer: Of course. Southern New Hampshire University and Arizona State University are examples.

Question: How about the opposite side of the coin? Do many schools survive that refuse to consider plans to reinvent themselves?

Answer: Yes, at least for schools that are top ranked or financially strong. Rollins College, with a large endowment, refused its president's request for substantial revision to its approach to education in 2011 and seems to be successful.

THE RISK PICTURE FOR UNIVERSITIES

By every indication, many universities need an enterprise risk management look at their ability to react to a disruption and take steps to convert from an unstable to a stable situation. The effort starts with a recognition of the total degree of risk. It involves a combination of both likelihood and size of potential loss.

- Severity: A negative event can be partial or total. It can be minor or serious.
- Frequency: A low frequency is a negative event that has rarely happened in the past or is not likely to occur in the future. A moderate frequency happens every so often. High frequency is reserved for events that occurred regularly and are likely in the near future.

Enterprise risk recognizes the likelihood that actual results will not match expected results.

- Variability: Expected results may not match predictions.
- Upside of risk: Results may be better or worse than expected.

From this perspective, some risks are serious and some are not. (See figure 4.1.)

- Minor loss: Would hurt but not be noticeable on financial statements; for example, a broken pipe in a student eating hall
- Significant loss: Causes a substantial impact on operations; for example, cancellation or delay by the government issuing visas for foreign exchange students
- Critical or major loss: Seriously hampers the ability to operate; for example, a fire that destroys a residence hall just before the start of semester
- Catastrophic loss: An unbearable financial loss causing an inability to continue operation; for example, a tornado that destroys facilities and equipment across the entire campus

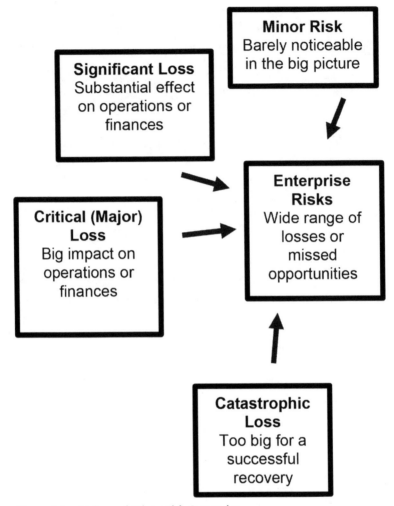

Figure 4.1. Major and Minor Risk Categories

Figure 4.2 shows how we recognize a progression of events when dealing with the differing impact of risks.

- Incident: An occurrence of seemingly minor importance that can lead to serious consequences if ignored
- Emergency: A serious situation when an incident demands immediate action to avoid more damage
- Crisis: A time of intense difficulty or danger; the quality and speed of the response determines the turning point for an improved or worse outcome
- Disaster: A point when the risk threatens the survival of the institution

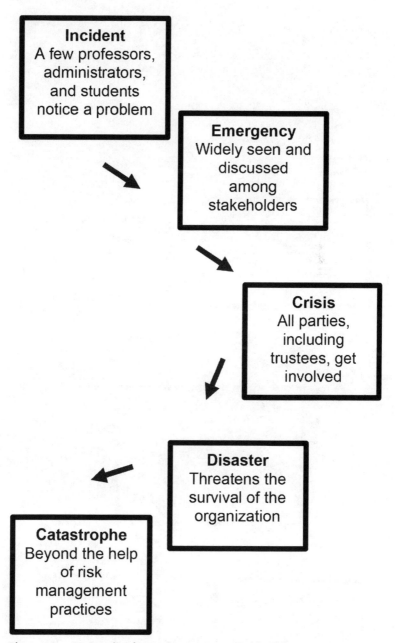

Figure 4.2. Progression from Minor to Catastrophic Risk

- Catastrophe: The final stage of organizational failure to deal with a risk; risk management efforts can rarely be effective at this level

EVALUATING RISK

Risk management creates systems to deal with negative events or missed opportunities. Figure 4.3 shows four of the activities.

- Prevention: Identify risk to be managed or opportunities to pursue and develop a strategy for addressing them.
- Detection: Identify conditions that reveal emerging risks or obstacles to achieving goals.

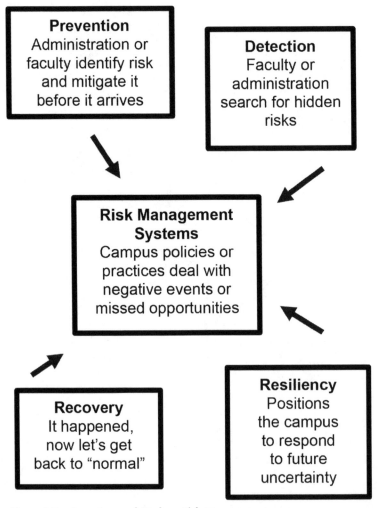

Figure 4.3.   Four Areas of Modern Risk Management

- Recovery: Address the risk condition or obstacle and attempt to eliminate it.
- Resilience: Either endure changing conditions or adapt new and successful behaviors in response to unexpected changes.

MANAGING RISK IN THE BUSINESS MODEL

From this foundation, we can assess the need for a more aggressive approach to risk management. Three situations are possible for a university:

- Mission and vision statement/no business model: The institution has been in business for a long time and has never linked its activities to a course of action that pursues long-term sustainable viability.
- Business model: The entity is struggling and talks about a business model and may be able to develop one before it merges or closes down.
- Urgency about a business model: The trustees and president recognize they are in trouble and are determined to make changes before it is too late.

Question: How many nonprofit colleges and universities are operating in the United States?
Answer: More than five thousand, if we count two-year and special purpose institutions. More than eighteen hundred private nonprofit and six hundred public entities offer bachelor's and/or master's degrees. More than six hundred are two-year public institutions offering associate degrees and certificates.

Question: How many are concerned that they should be pursuing a new business model with some urgency?
Answer: By all indications, not a high percentage.

Question: How many should be concerned that time may run out if they do not develop a new business model?
Answer: We need to provide a framework for answering this question.

INSTITUTIONAL CATEGORY

Colleges and universities have markedly different conditions that shape their environment. A first step in developing a business model is to acknowledge the institutional position in the Carnegie Classification of Institutions of Higher Education:

- Doctoral universities: Award twenty or more research/scholarship or professional practice doctoral degrees annually; alternatively, consider themselves to be research universities
- Master's colleges and universities: Award fifty or more master's degrees annually
- Baccalaureate colleges: More than half of degrees are baccalaureate or master's level; divided into subcategories as arts and sciences focus or diverse fields
- Baccalaureate/associate colleges: More than half of degrees are associates level
- Associate's colleges: Highest degree awarded is an associate's degree
- Special focus institutions: Business, law, healthcare, technical, engineering, and more
- Tribal colleges: Members of the American Indian Higher Education Consortium

Question: Why does a university have to acknowledge its Carnegie category?
Answer: It helps a school be realistic about its programs, markets, and capability to achieve success.

Question: Don't most schools know this already?
Answer: Not really. Some master's institutions think they are research institutions. For that matter, even many baccalaureate entities act the same way.

FINANCIAL HEALTH

A university can further be matched to a classification based upon financial strength. This can be measured by factors such as tuition dependency, endowment income, assets, debt, and other financial health measures. These measures can give us a useful perspective for comparisons. In terms of financial status, three categories emerge:

- Well-endowed school with respected reputation: It can deliver whatever it wants to whomever it pleases at whatever price it wants to charge. These institutions barely noticed the 2020 Coronavirus pandemic as they know they can rely upon an unchallengeable financial position and reputation.
- Poorly endowed school with respected reputation: It struggles to find students who want its degree and will pay to get it. The school hopes it can survive by figuring out how to solve a declining financial position before its potential students recognize its problems.

- Poorly endowed school known only locally: It often has no clue how it can continue to deliver an education to students who do not seem to want its degrees and who cannot or will not pay for them at a price that gives the school a good chance to survive.

To identify the financial health category for a university, separate from reputation, we can check the *Forbes'* College Financial Health Grades. These are reported periodically for the better-known private not-for-profit colleges in the United States with enrollments greater than five hundred students. *Forbes* evaluates financial strength based on factors such as the institution's assets, debt, and operating and benefactor cash flow. Table 4.2 shows the picture in a recent year. Figure 4.4 contains another view.

Table 4.2. *Forbes'* College Financial Health Grades

Financial Grade 2019	Number of Schools	Percent of Total
A+	34	4%
A	21	2%
A-	19	2%
B+	47	5%
B	52	6%
B-	85	9%
C+	166	18%
C	184	19%
C-	148	16%
D	177	19%
Total	933	100%

We now have a more complete picture to answer questions about the urgency of assessing the viability of the model.

- Institutional category: Schools in any of the categories may need to examine their business model.
- Endowment level: Well-endowed schools may have a less urgent need to review their viability than lesser-endowed institutions, or the endowment alone may be misleading.

The overall financial health picture, as reflected in the *Forbes* ranking, is likely the best indication of the level of urgency for reviewing the business model. Simply ranked:

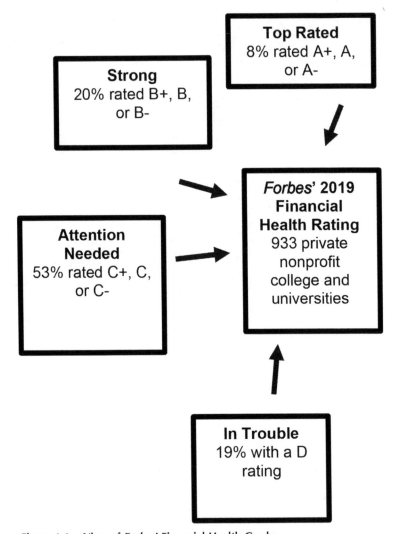

Figure 4.4.   View of *Forbes'* Financial Health Grades

- A grade: The institution has maximum flexibility to work with its current business model and should make changes consistent with good management practices.
- B grade: The institution has a little more urgency to review its activities but probably does not need a major overall of the business model.
- C grade: The institution definitely needs to review the long-term financial sustainability of its business model.

- D grade: The institution needs a sense of urgency about the viability of its business model.

CONCLUSION

For well-endowed or other financially stable universities, the business model should be reviewed periodically. Also, new planning measures should monitor viability of their missions, visions, and values. For universities hovering near or actually facing serious financial difficulty, a more urgent approach is strongly recommended.

Chapter Five

How Does a University Revise Its Business Model? Are We Getting into the World of Business Continuity Planning?

BUSINESS CONTINUITY

Business continuity planning is the process of identifying steps to respond to disruption, manage short-term challenges, recover a stable operating position, and resume a stable level of operation. The process is undertaken by one or more groups assigned to create the plan.

A business continuity plan (BCP) is a formal process of evaluating risk and proposing how to manage it. It identifies current activities and opportunities and develops a strategy to ensure the institution is operating efficiently. This includes designing and delivering academic products or services, identifying target markets, and delivering services on a sustainable financial foundation.

Question: What is the biggest risk associated with business continuity planning in a college or university?
Answer: It's the failure to understand the scope of the effort.

- Internal scope: It's not about what we are doing. It's about what we need to do.
- External scope: It's not about what others are doing so we can copy them. It's about what we should do based on our own capabilities and resources.

The goal and scope of a business continuity plan is simple. Figure 5.1 shows the goal of the process is to create a financially sustainable model.

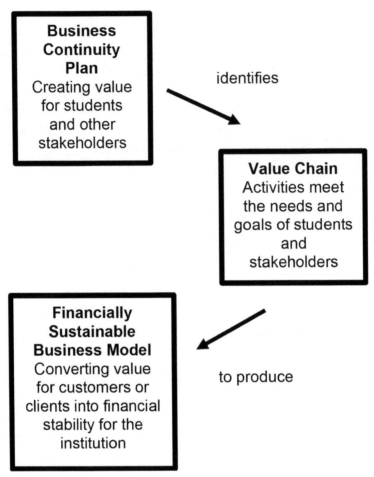

Figure 5.1. Scope of a University Business Continuity Plan

BUSINESS CONTINUITY PLAN (BCP) TASK FORCE

A task force is a group of individuals identified to pursue a single temporary goal. Generically, a task force addresses problems or practices that do not have attention from various units in an organization. As a result of the lack of coordinated attention to a specific risk, the university is in danger of failing to prepare itself for sustained long-term continuity.

An organization can begin continuity planning with the formation of a multiple task forces. The goal is to create and share business continuity plans and consolidate and coordinate recommendations into a single BCP. Figure 5.2 shows possible directives to each task force.

- Task definition: Bring a recommendation to the president in the form of a plan to pursue long-term sustainable viability of the institution.
- Target date: Specify the desired date for submitting the report containing the continuity plan.
- Membership: Identify the task force leader and members, likely to be administrators, faculty members, and representatives of the president and trustees.
- Focus: Ask the task force to prepare a recommendation that takes a holistic view of the future rather than a retrospective view of what we are doing or what we have done.

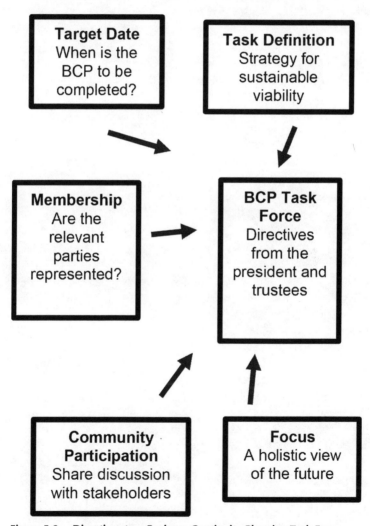

Figure 5.2. Directives to a Business Continuity Planning Task Force

- Community participation: Ask the task force to communicate and share progress with university stakeholders (faculty, students, administrators, other staff, and external alumni).

The function of a task force is solely to achieve a single goal. The membership of the task force often determines whether the goal will be achieved.

Creating a business model and value chain usually brings together multiple viewpoints. In this sense, the team should be composed of people with different interests and skills.

Task force members also should be people who are willing to listen to others who have different perspectives. Individual members should be seeking solutions to problems even when they do not get their own way.

Question: Is a BCP task force also a team?
Answer: Maybe yes, maybe no. It depends on your definition of a team.

Question: What are some definitions of a team?
Answer:

- A group of players forming one side in a competitive game or sport
- A group with a single focus—to win
- Individuals who join together to achieve a common goal

A poor business model and weak value chain is a losing situation. Teams do not form easily under such circumstances.

A university needs to recognize the characteristics of effective teams when they address business continuity. Figure 5.3 identifies desirable characteristics of members of the task force.

- Problem solver: Understands the raison d'être and wants to be a part of finding solutions to perceived problems
- Reliable "player": Meets commitments and follows through on assignments; members need to depend on each other
- Effective communicator: Expresses thoughts and ideas clearly, honestly, and with respect for others in a positive, yet confident, and respectful manner
- Active listener: Absorbs, reflects upon, and seeks to understand ideas, particularly those that arise from different points of view
- Active, not defensive, discussant: Not prone to quick reactions resembling debate or argument; teams need dialogue, not confrontation, when new ideas are developed

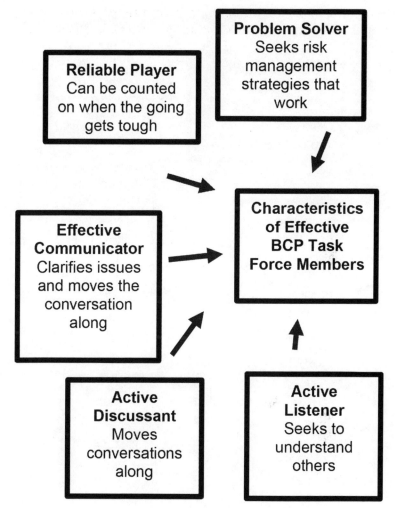

Figure 5.3. Desirable Characteristics of BCP Task Force Members

Additionally, figure 5.4 lists certain behaviors that are sought from selected members.

- Helps others: Shares ideas, information, knowledge, and personal experiences to improve suggestions or proposals of others
- Cooperates on group tasks: Pitches in to perform tasks, particularly when initiative is needed or others seek assistance
- Exhibits flexible behavior: Adapts to changing roles or conditions without exhibiting signs of or behavior showing of stress or anger

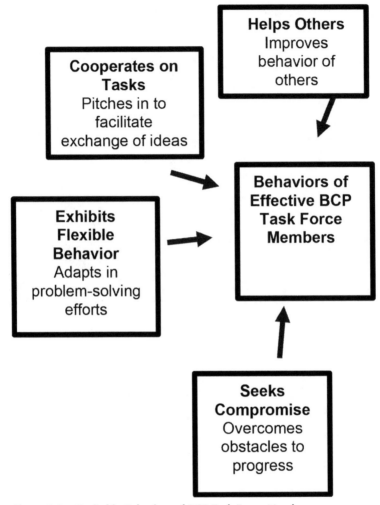

Figure 5.4.   Desirable Behaviors of BCP Task Force Members

- Seeks compromise: Doesn't "lock down" or exhibit rigid behavior that blocks forward movement

It may seem obvious that a BCP team should be composed of individuals with these characteristics and expected behaviors. In fact, universities have two broad choices for forming teams in a BCP process:

- Bureaucratic team: Reflects the organizational hierarchy
- Innovative team: Recognizes the urgency of seeking new ideas and change

Figure 5.5 shows an example of a bureaucratic team.

BUREAUCRATIC TEAM

A bureaucratic team reflects a hierarchical structure with specialized units, rules and regulations defining authority and power, formal job descriptions, impersonal decision making, and limited empathy to people or duties.

Universities often ignore the personal characteristics of effective team members when they form task forces to deal with real problems. They seek representation by a formula that does not consider the skills needed for

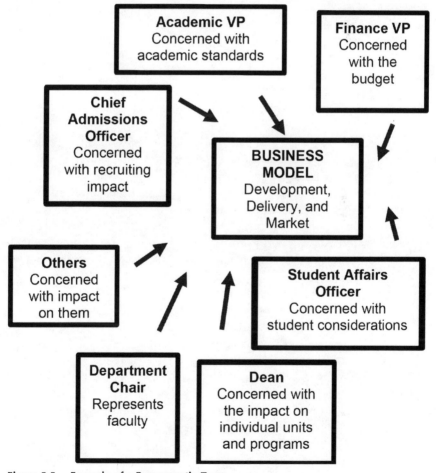

Figure 5.5. Example of a Bureaucratic Team

problem solving. Instead, the task force is composed of individuals who do not see the big picture and are not vetted against the characteristics of good team players.

Question: So what happens to the task force?
Answer: It is composed of someone from the offices of vice presidents or deans, professors from various academic units, and other stray administrators.

Question: What's the problem with that?
Answer: Members see the task as representing their home unit as opposed to solving real problems. They may even disagree that a problem exists. The success rate of bureaucratic teams to form an effective business model is not high.

Question: Will a bureaucracy support a recommendation to pursue innovation and participate in making it happen?
Answer: Yes. Bureaucracies totally support change as long as nothing is different in their daily work lives.

INNOVATIVE TEAM

The innovative team has a membership in stark contrast to the bureaucratic model. Its members are selected as an exception to the stability and equilibrium goals of a bureaucracy. Key players are not chosen based solely on credentials and position titles; they are evaluated by their motivations and behavior. Figure 5.6 shows potential members.

- Team leader: Has the motivation, authority, and power to interact with the group to propose and implement a new business model in an outdated academic environment
- Entrepreneur: Seeks to do something different that builds a business model around unmet needs and consistent with changing markets
- Conscientious entrepreneur: Argues for change that is accompanied by positive social and economic benefits
- Intrapreneur: Brings the latest technology to the discussion
- Investor: Ensures that the model adequately includes the components to deliver the proposed outcomes on a sustainable financial foundation

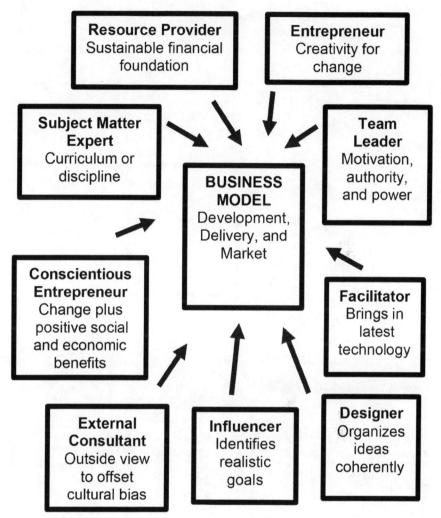

Figure 5.6. Example of an Innovative Team

- Designer: Brings ideas together into a coherent package to share with others
- External consultant: Brings in an outside view and an offset to cultural bias

Figure 5.7 provides a way to look at the innovative team in terms of specific concepts that fit the members.

- The manager: Provides the team with a leader, which is always needed
- The brain: Has a broad knowledge, problem-solving focus, and a natural sense for blending complex issues into risk management solutions

- The visionary: Sees the big picture and is creative with strategies for pursuing future opportunities
- The strategist: Identifies risks and opportunities and matches them with options
- The salesman: Focuses on customer needs and matches them with powerful messages to drive the value chain
- The technology guru: Understands intricacies of technology needed to build a powerful communications strategy

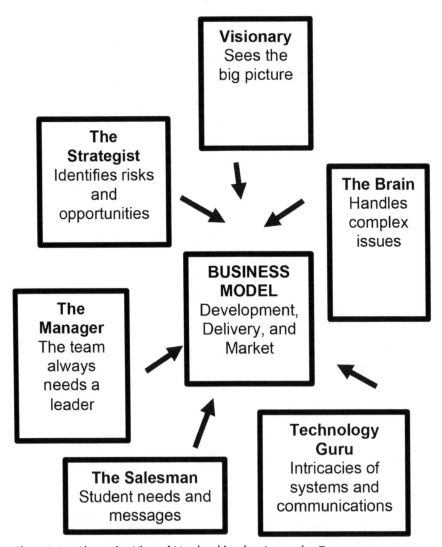

Figure 5.7.   Alternative View of Membership of an Innovative Team

CONCLUSION

This finishes a discussion on the framework of a business continuity plan task force. In the sense of finding a workable solution to the challenges facing our university, we move on to specific business models and examine them in the context of business continuity planning.

Chapter Six

Where Does the Liberal Arts Fit in a Sustainable Value Chain for a University? Does Anyone Really Care about Shakespeare?

Question: What on earth does it mean to "throw in the towel"?

Answer: It occurs when a manager can no longer watch the carnage being inflicted on his boxer. He throws a towel into the boxing ring to indicate surrender. Younger people, particularly those who did not grow up watching Sylvester Stallone in the *Rocky* movies, may not be familiar with the term.

Absent such outside factors as a loss of electricity, a boxing match can end in one of four ways:

- Knockout: One boxer has been knocked down and is unable to rise and resume boxing within a specified time.
- Fight is stopped without a knockout: After a fixed period of time, both fighters are standing, so judges or the referee declare a winner and loser.
- Draw: The fight ends with neither party declared the winner or loser.
- One party quits: The boxer or manager of the boxer concedes the fight.

In many ways, private nonprofit colleges have been waging a boxing match. Many of them have been hammered by their competitors and even spectators.

Question: Which is the likely outcome for a lesser-endowed private college or university in the current battles for dominance in higher education?

A. A knockout
B. A draw
C. One party quits
D. The fight ends with all parties standing

Answer: D. The fight ends with all parties standing. No one wins with knock-outs, draws, or quitting the battle.

Thus, the innovative business continuity task force has the goal of avoiding a knockout or worse. To do so, many universities need tuition-paying students. Let's start with them in our effort to identify issues and develop strategies to shape or reshape the business model and value chain.

A FOCUS ON OUR STUDENTS

We know who we want as our students. We know what we hope they will learn. The challenge is to find and educate them. If we do a good job creating successful graduates, we will also be creating a reputation that brings future students (customers) to the institution.

To attract students, a university initially engages parents, students, or other adults and asks them to make a purchase. The potential student seeks knowledge and skills. The university converts the student into something more useful for society. In this context, the business continuity task force recognizes the three roles of students shown in figure 6.1.

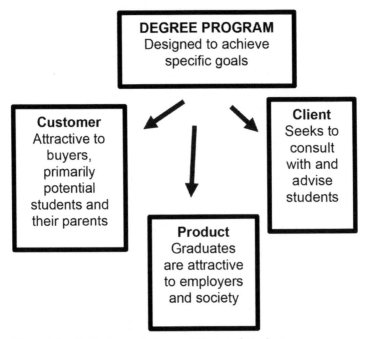

Figure 6.1.   **Student as a Customer, Client, and Product**

- Customer: Someone has to buy the "product" of the university. It may be the student, a parent, or a third party who encourages or even finances a college education.
- Client: Once a purchase is made, the student becomes a client in the sense of using the services of the institution. It is not enough to sell admission. The institution must support the effort to graduate.
- Product: Once graduated, the alumnus spreads the word of the value of the education. The graduate is a product in that sense that the university created a skilled and knowledgeable citizen of the community.

WHAT DO OUR STUDENTS WANT?

Next, we ask, "What do our students want?" Figure 6.2 shows that the value of the right university degree comes from specific outcomes, including the following:

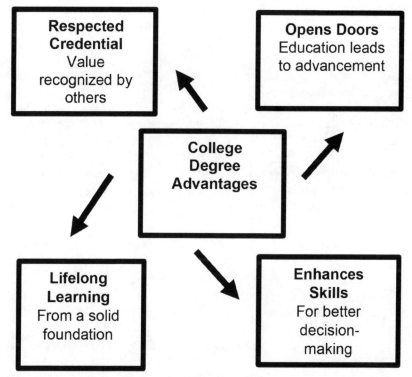

Figure 6.2.   Values Associated with College Degrees

- Provides a respected credential: A bachelor's degree is an expectation, and often a requirement, to find employment in many organizations and fields of endeavor. An MBA enhances the recognition.
- Opens doors: Degrees are a key factor in hiring decisions by corporations, nonprofits, and government agencies.
- Enhances decision-making skills: Education develops critical thinking, problem-solving skills, and cultural, ethical, political, and economic understanding.
- Encourages lifelong learning: Personal and professional values adjust over a lifetime of experiences. A master's degree adds a level of renewal after completing a bachelor's degree and a variety of adult experiences and activities. For some individuals, a post-master's degree adds problem-solving skills needed for complex decision making.

WHAT DO OUR STUDENTS NEED?

The unique value of a liberal arts–based college experience is that it develops an understanding of decision making for adult life: Essentially, problem solving occurs in four areas as shown in figure 6.3.

- Solving problems involving discovery: Advance knowledge of risk management processes
- Solving problems involving integration: Synthesize information across disciplines or time periods; create new patterns or expand knowledge into new contexts

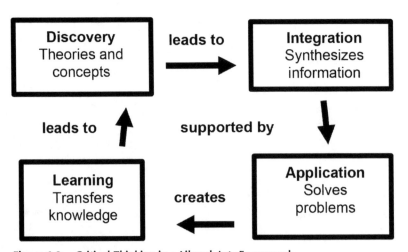

Figure 6.3.   Critical Thinking in a Liberal Arts Framework

- Solving problems involving application: Advance knowledge to augment prior research or solve problems; undertake collaboration and evaluation by peers and other parties
- Solving problems involving learning: Improve the transfer of knowledge from teacher or mentor to student or facilitate learning

DOES THE TRADITIONAL COLLEGE MODEL SUPPORT CRITICAL THINKING?

Although we have widespread agreement that the liberal arts provides valuable learning outcomes, the traditional model is not optimal to produce them. As shown in figure 6.4, it deals with issues that are obstacles to curriculum reform on many campuses.

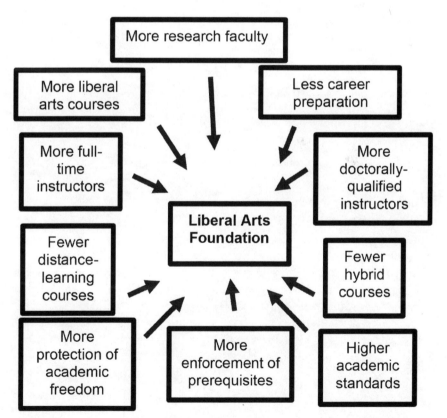

Figure 6.4. Common Demands That Do Not Improve a Liberal Arts Foundation to a Curriculum

Table 6.1 is a self-test of a person's own view of the traditional model of the liberal arts core for a university.

Table 6.1. Quiz on Reform of the Traditional Liberal Arts Core

Circle the number that matches strongly agree, agree, neutral, disagree, or strongly disagree. A high total score means you are comfortable with a traditional model. With a low score, you are an advocate for change.

	SA	A	N	D	SD
1. Colleges should require more mandatory liberal arts courses.	10	8	6	4	2
2. Colleges should offer fewer career preparation (internships, cooperative education) courses.	10	8	6	4	2
3. Colleges should seek or maintain a high percentage of full-time (not part-time) professors on the faculty.	10	8	6	4	2
4. Colleges should seek or maintain a high percentage of doctorally qualified professors on the faculty.	10	8	6	4	2
5. Colleges should seek or maintain a high percentage of professors engaged in academic scholarship.	10	8	6	4	2
6. Colleges should offer few, if any, distance-learning courses at the undergraduate level.	10	8	6	4	2
7. Colleges should offer few, if any, hybrid courses at the undergraduate level.	10	8	6	4	2
8. Colleges should provide more protection for academic freedom.	10	8	6	4	2
9. Colleges should insist on stronger enforcement of prerequisites.	10	8	6	4	2
10. Colleges should implement more stringent rules for graduation.	10	8	6	4	2

LIBERAL ARTS CORE OUTCOMES

Let's take a look at a serious reform of the liberal arts foundation in the framework of a four-year college degree. Figure 6.5 shows that the liberal arts foundation seeks learning outcomes in two categories of intellectual and practical skills, personal and social responsibility, local and global civic engagement, intercultural knowledge and competence, ethical reasoning, and skills for lifelong and global learning.

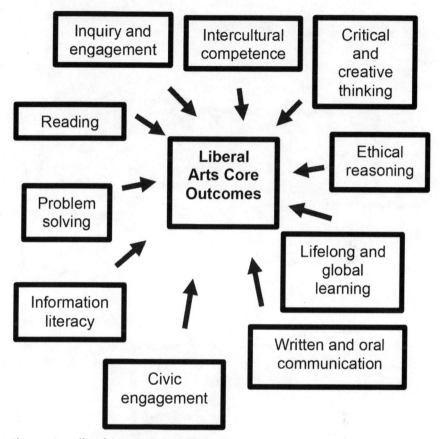

Figure 6.5.   Liberal Arts Core Outcomes

BACHELOR'S DEGREE OUTCOMES

Whatever the specific motives, liberal arts sets up the expectations and outcomes from any college curriculum that requires the foundation. Across all forms of intelligence and STEM (science, technology, engineering, mathematics) and non-STEM curriculums, professors seek to increase the likelihood that students will be prepared to pursue sustainable financial and social success. Basically, this is a four-part structure of learning outcomes, as shown in figure 6.6.

- Improved written and oral communications skills
- A better understanding of ethical responsibilities
- A better understanding of strategic thinking
- Enhanced ability to reason analytically and make data-driven decisions

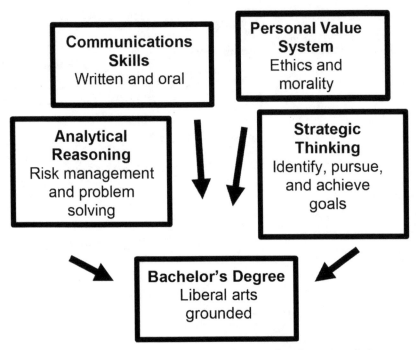

Figure 6.6.   Bachelor's Degree Outcomes Built on a Liberal Arts Foundation

LIBERAL ARTS CORE COURSES

The liberal arts outcomes require a minimum number of courses to achieve diversity of viewpoints and coverage of foundation concepts. In the traditional model, the liberal arts courses are mixed with general education courses in a model that may account for half the courses in a four-year degree program.

Professors often have firm views of the value of the courses in their own academic areas. This can lead to relatively inflexible curriculum designs where an academic core resembles distributive requirements more than a serious effort to achieve liberal arts outcomes. Thirty credit hours, ten courses representing 3 credit hours each, is often viewed as a minimal-sized core by independent observers. As an example, it might be designed with topics like those shown in table 6.2.

Table 6.2.   Example of 30-Credit Liberal Arts Core

	Credits
Area 1. Communication	3
Area 2. Arts and Humanities	6
Area 3. History	3
Area 4. Social and Behavioral Sciences	6
Area 5. Physical and Life Sciences	6
Area 6. International Studies	3
Area 7. Ethics and Values	3
Total	30

Figure 6.7 illustrates this structure.

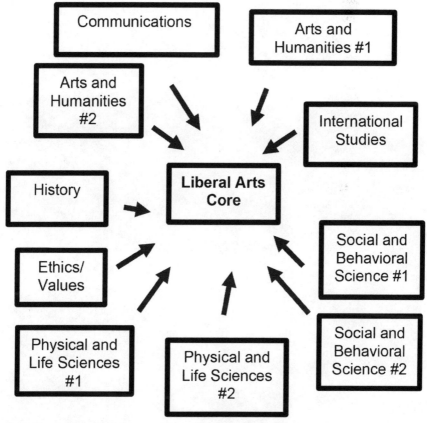

Figure 6.7.   Liberal Arts Core with 30 Credits in Eight Areas

CONCLUSION

For the purposes of business continuity, we can dismiss critics who claim obsolescence or other failures of the liberal arts. A college degree may not be a goal for everyone, but the liberal arts is certainly a strong foundation for an educated human being.

At the same time, liberal arts colleges have a business continuity shortcoming with respect to the traditional academic model. Let's take a look at a pathway to correcting it while retaining the liberal arts foundation.

Chapter Seven

Business Continuity Plan on a Liberal Arts Foundation: What Do We Have to Consider? What Do We Have to Change?

BUSINESS MODEL AND PHILOSOPHY

Business continuity planning starts with a business model. We will work with the following:

- We offer undergraduate degrees and courses in traditional, remote, hybrid, and/or distance-learning formats and match student needs with programs that create or continue a financially sustainable institution.

We add to it our educational philosophy. Today's highly competitive environment in higher education demands a focus on the structure and delivery of degree programs. The concepts come together in the need to join critical thinking and career preparation in packages that meet different needs of a diverse field of high school graduates and adult learners. These programs and courses reflect new and more effective outcomes from higher education. The approaches deliver improved learning outcomes based on their curriculum designs, course formats, and the availability of personal student choices. They are sufficiently attractive so as to be financially sustainable.

Figure 7.1 addresses these issues. Figure 7.2 shows the business model supported by a value chain.

- Solid product: Relevant and valuable degrees to meet student goals
- High-quality design: Relevant courses and support services
- Flexible delivery: Hybrid, remote, and distance-learning formats

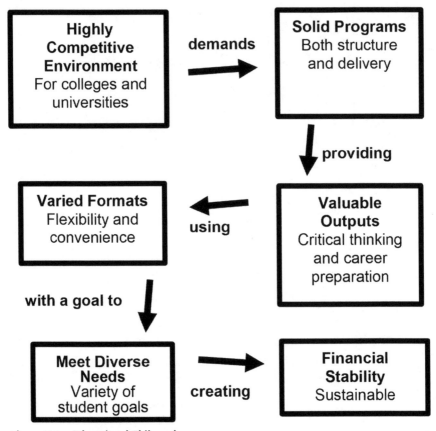

Figure 7.1.   Educational Philosophy

- Motivated customers: Parents and students seeking respected degrees
- Financial sustainability: Positive long-term cash flow picture
- Program outcome: Graduates with valuable new knowledge and skills

VALUE CHAIN ANALYSIS—STUDENT COMPONENT

In the framework of a business model, we conduct a value chain analysis. We already asked what students need from a liberal arts core. Now we ask, "Who are the students?" The answer creates the picture of our target market. It also answers two other questions: Who should pay for college? Why would they be willing to pay?

Figure 7.3 is one way to identify and segment an undergraduate student population.

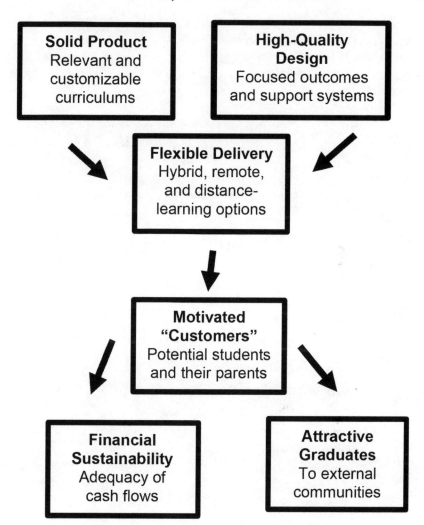

Figure 7.2. Business Model and Value Chain for a Degree Program

- Full-time residential students: Young adults eighteen to twenty-five years of age who enroll directly or after a gap year from high school, attend full-time, and do not have major life and work responsibilities like dependents and full-time jobs; also known as traditional students
- Full-time commuter students: Same characteristics as traditional students except for living in university housing
- Nontraditional students: Adult learners older than the age of twenty-five who have major life and work responsibilities

- International students: Enrolled for credit at an accredited higher education institution in the United States on a temporary visa
- Other student classifications: Include first-generation college students, non-native speakers of English, students with disabilities, and working students

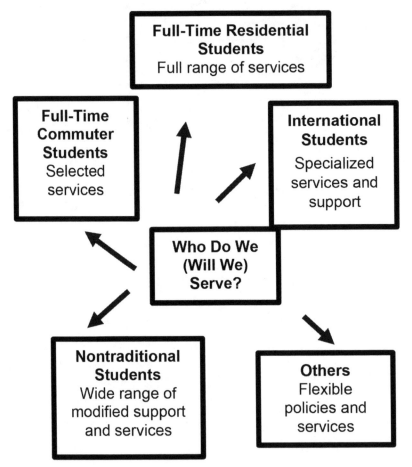

Figure 7.3.   Categories of Undergraduate Students

WHAT FACTORS SHAPE STUDENT CHOICES OF COLLEGES?

We know what we are doing today. Is it what our students want? Figure 7.4 shows an assessment of students and their needs and goals.

- Timing of college: Some students attend immediately after graduation from high school. Some undertake a short delay. Others may take a long delay or quit, only to return years later to finish school.

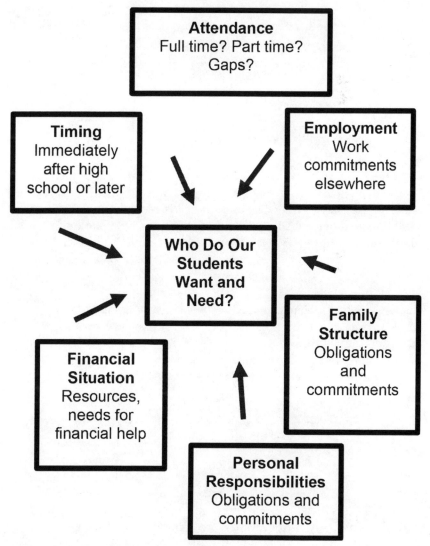

Figure 7.4. Factors Shaping College Choice

- Full-time or part-time attendance: Some students are committed to three or more years of full-time pursuit of a degree. Some are not.
- Employment: Some students have serious paid-work responsibilities that support or interfere with college courses.
- Financial situation: Family income or wealth eases the cost of college for some students. The lack of such resources must be overcome for others.
- Family structure: Some students live with parents in a family structure and can return home every day or even at the end of a class term. Some do not.
- Personal responsibilities: Some students only have to worry about themselves. Others have family or health issues, are supporting dependents, or are dealing with other commitments that distract them from their education.
- Prior education: Some are well prepared from their background in high school or time spent in another college before transferring. Others need help adjusting to college expectations and requirements.

WHAT FACTORS MOTIVATE STUDENTS TO ATTEND COLLEGE?

A question that might be asked by the business continuity planning team is, "Do we know what students are searching for when they choose a college?" We know they have a full range of goals and concerns. What is important to a full-time traditional residential student may be of little interest to a single parent working full-time to earn enough money to raise a small child.

Table 7.1 shows ten of the more than fifty motives for attending college. How important is each one to each category of student?

Question: What is the meaning of the total score in the figure?
Answer: Since the total possible score is 10, average scores near 5 reflect many unimportant factors. This is not a surprise. Few students or parents get everything they want out of a college. A business continuity plan attempts to identify the most important factors and offer as many of them as fits the plan.

ACADEMIC MOTIVES FOR ATTENDING COLLEGE

Separately from their practical motives, many students pursue their interests—and hence colleges—based on their personal capabilities and desired use of time. These factors match the ten categories of intelligence. Students possessing skills resulting from one or more forms of intelligence are likely to choose a college that affords them the opportunity to display those skills.

Table 7.1. Possible Scores on Importance of Factors for Three Categories of Students

		Age 17 Full-time Residential Student	Age 25 Part-time Working Commuter	Age 30 Part-time Working Parent
1	More qualified for a job	5	8	6
2	Make more money	6	7	9
3	Improve social network	6	4	2
4	Get a college degree	8	10	10
5	Find my career direction	8	4	2
6	Free time on weekends	6	2	1
7	Fix bad prior decision	1	6	8
8	Skills for retirement	2	2	2
9	Reinvent myself	2	8	6
10	Find mentor or advisers	7	4	2
	Average score	5.1	5.5	4.8

Note: 10 = highest, 1 = lowest, maximum score is 100.

Figure 7.5 shows the ten forms of intelligence that affect choice of institutions and programs.

- Situational: Students are capable of participating in different settings and can work successfully in a wide range of college experiences.
- Musical: Students seek to include music, either as a possible career field or at least as a component of the college experience.
- Logical: Students have been successful in high school courses because of their ability to perceive relationships, make connections among data elements, and use sequential reasoning skills. These students seek academic challenge.
- Mathematical: The ability to calculate, quantify, and understand and use numbers leads students to STEM (science, technology, engineering, or mathematics) programs.
- Existential: The capacity and interest to tackle deep questions about human existence produces a desire to go to a school with opportunities to do research.
- Interpersonal: The ability to understand and interact effectively with others adds a strong social component to the choice of a college.
- Bodily: Physical and athletic skills lead students to schools where they can demonstrate them in sports and related activities.
- Linguistic: The ability to use language to express and appreciate complex meanings leads students to choose language and communications programs.

- Introspective: Capacity to understand their own thoughts, feelings, strengths, and weaknesses can lead students to many different places for a college-level education.
- Spatial: The ability to use their imagination to manipulate images and understand graphics can lead students to design and art programs.

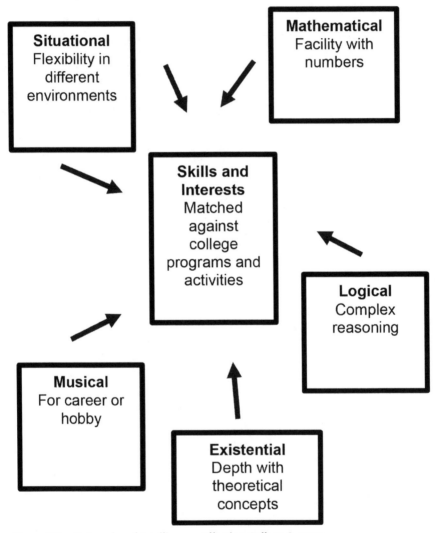

Figure 7.5.   Categories of Intelligence Affecting College Success

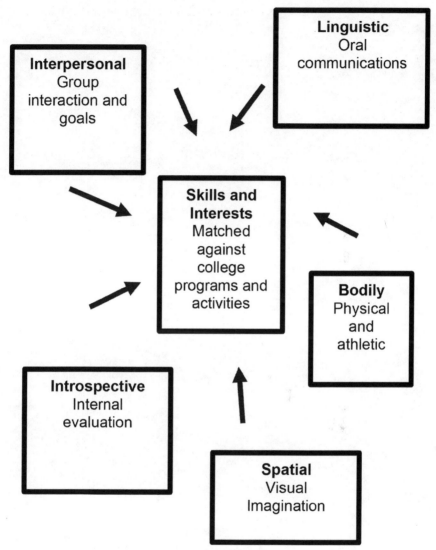

Figure 7.5. Categories of Intelligence Affecting College Success (continued)

CONCLUSION

Our value chain analysis starts with potential markets for academic programs and services. It creates a direction for us to design our products with characteristics that motivate applications from parents and financial support from parents and others. Next, we move to the issues of designing our product.

Chapter Eight

Let's Build a Modern Curriculum on a Liberal Arts Foundation: Hey, This Is a Program That Really Meets My Needs!

CURRICULUM DESIGN

The business continuity problem is not the liberal arts core. Rather, it may occur from a failure to differentiate the difference between a liberal arts foundation and the application of liberal arts outcomes to careers and courses of action after graduation from college.

In this framework, a non-STEM degree can be designed to give flexibility in three areas, as shown in figure 8.1.

- Liberal arts foundation: Develops the intellectual and practical skills and a value system built upon personal and social responsibility
- Liberal arts and/or career-oriented major: Adds depth, enhancing knowledge and problem-solving capabilities
- Electives: Offer the opportunity to enrich a person with study in areas not necessarily tied to the curriculum expectations of educators or others

DESIGN OF A COLLEGE PROGRAM

The business value chain for a specific academic program needs a high-quality product where students learn skills that help them be successful as adults. Figure 8.2 shows elements in the design of effective degree programs.

- Clear objectives: An explanation of the goals to be achieved by graduates from a program
- High expectations: Clear messages that respond to the situation of potential students and their families

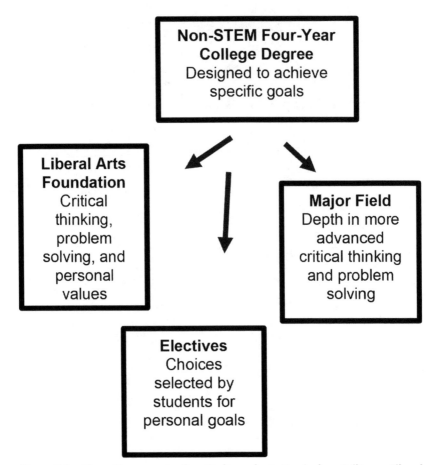

Figure 8.1.   Three Components of an Undergraduate Curriculum Built on a Liberal Arts Foundation

- Value formulation: Inherent features that encourage behaviors consistent with successful behaviors with interacting with others
- Relevance: A design to maximize the benefits from new ideas and technology
- Expansive knowledge: A wide area of critical thinking in terms of the value of individual courses in the learning experience
- Tailorable: Flexibility for students, professors, and advisers to modify courses to cultivate unique skills and educational experiences

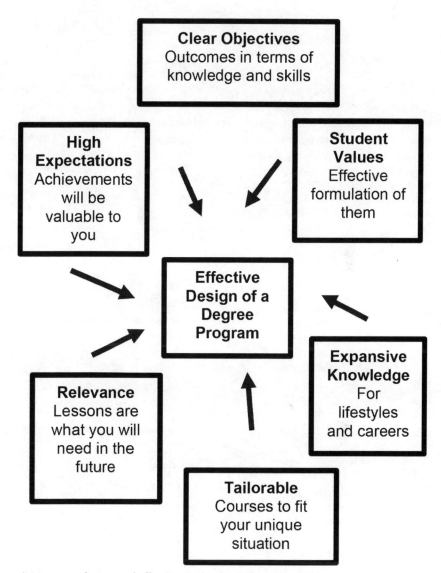

Figure 8.2. Elements of Effective Design for College Programs

COLLEGE COURSE FORMATS

Once the content has been determined, the institution identifies the specific formats for course delivery. Figure 8.3 shows the primary choices.

- Lecture: Instructor presents material orally or via video followed by discussion and evaluating outcomes.
- Blended learning: Material is studied or practiced outside the class setting
  and students join the instructor to discuss the learning points.
- Distance learning: Material is studied and evaluated individually without
  regular interaction with an instructor.
- Remote learning: Structured as blended learning, instructor and student
  interaction occurs with the aid of video conferencing software. Students
  join class sessions via a webcam or smart phone. Professors and students
  are able to see and talk to each other The instructor can share instructional
  materials on the computer screen.

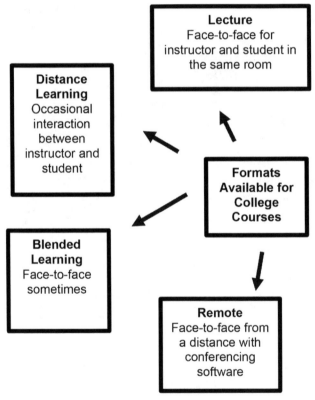

Figure 8.3.   Formats of College Courses

Question: Of lecture, distance learning, blended learning, and remote learning, which is preferred by instructors and students?
Answer: The answer depends upon the individual situation, including the skill of the instructor and goals and needs of the student.

FLEXIBLE FORMATS OF COURSES

The formatting possibilities (lecture, distance learning, blended, remote) offer the student and institution maximum flexibility as the design for a college course. For each three-credit course:

- Lecture: Student attends twenty to twenty-four classroom sessions.
- Blended: Student attends ten to twenty classroom sessions and completes asynchronous activities to replace in-person sessions.
- Remote: Student attends ten to twenty Zoom-style sessions replacing the classroom sessions.
- Online: Student takes the class asynchronously.

EVALUATION OF STUDENT PERFORMANCE

In all formats, grading is based on measurements suitable to the academic discipline. Let's suppose this would be a midterm and final written exam/assignment covering material in a syllabus, textbook, other references or distributed materials, and asynchronous videos. Grading variations include

- Lecture: A mid-term and final exam/assignment, as found in the traditional model
- Distance: A third written submission required to cover learning outcomes in the traditional model
- Blended or remote: An extra written submission required covering the individual assignments replacing traditional attendance

Figure 8.4 shows this evaluation structure.

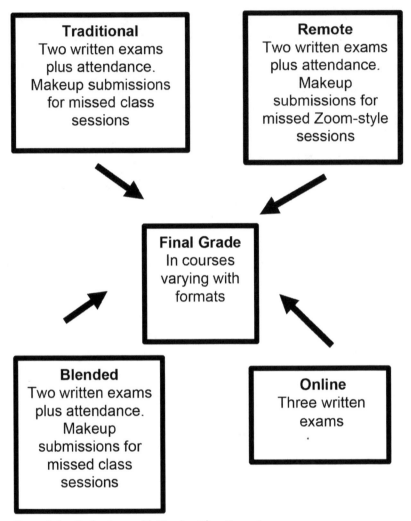

Figure 8.4. Evaluations with Varying Class Formats

CONCLUSION

The framework for business continuity planning demands an understanding of what a college is doing and what it seeks to do better. Absent this foundation, colleges may find themselves out of touch with the needs of students and the realities of higher education. The goal of BCP is to ensure that the activities are built upon a value chain that will ensure the institution's own success in the future.

Chapter Nine

Let's Build Our Own Undergraduate Degree on a Liberal Arts Foundation: If We Design and Offer the Right Products, Will They Come?

A UNIQUE COLLEGE EXPERIENCE

We are now ready to create a new model for an undergraduate degree. We will build it on a foundation of 120 to 126 credit hours leading to one or two degrees matching the following principles:

- Past experience of student: Full credit for prior college-level courses
- Goals of student: Thirty-credit-hour blocs of courses allowing students to pursue customized learning outcomes matched to their goals

Students choose to pursue one or more degrees, specifically:

- BS in liberal arts .... 120 credits
- BS in business administration .... 120 credits
- Two BS degrees: liberal arts and business administration   120 credits
- MBA alone. .... 36 credits
- Dual Degree: BS and MBA .... 126 credits

RECRUITING MESSAGE

Our program can be described succinctly to students, parents, employers, and high school counselors as follows:

- The program offers students the best of both worlds: the highly valued liberal arts foundation and the advantages of career preparation. Faculty advisers work with students to create an individualized curriculum to meet a student's goals and needs.

ADMISSION REQUIREMENTS

We can also provide a statement of the admission philosophies.

- Bachelor's degree or dual degrees: A high school diploma or other evidence of ability to engage successfully with college-level topics and requirements
- Master of business administration: A college or university diploma or other evidence of ability to engage successfully with graduate-level topics and requirements

This can be followed by providing more information, such as the following:

- Credit request for prior coursework: Advanced high school courses and courses from other accredited colleges up to a limit of 75 credit hours
- Transcripts verifying prior course work: Official or unofficial copies required
- Degree desired: A statement of the student's academic goal

GRADUATION FLEXIBILITY

The program can offer flexibility and assurances in its details. Examples include the following:

- Specific liberal arts major: If 24 upper-division liberal arts or business credits are taken in a single discipline, the liberal arts degree converts to that major program.
- Commitment to students: Transfer students who follow an approved program are guaranteed a program design limit of 120 credits. The university could also confirm that the entire degree would be available in a specific format (blended, remote, distance learning).

COURSE FORMATS

The format for courses is remote learning using conferencing software such as Zoom. Some classes may offer options that include traditional classroom and total distance learning.

COMPETITIVE TUITION

A candidate makes a tuition payment as part of registration for each course.

COURSE SCHEDULE

Figure 9.1 shows classes offered starting in September, December, March, or June. The program is self-paced. Accepted candidates can register for a term or skip a term.

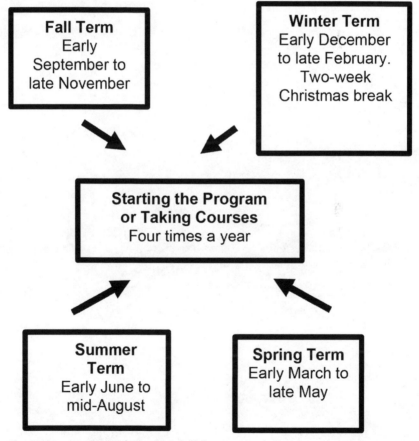

Figure 9.1.   Year-Round Course Schedule

COURSES AND CURRICULUMS

Table 9.1 provides an overview of options available to students:

Table 9.1. Major Components of the Curriculum

Area	Credits
Liberal Arts Foundation. Expands the capacity of the mind to think critically and analyze information effectively. May be zero for transfer students.	30
Liberal Arts Major Area. Allows exploration of ideas and a deeper understanding of a single area of academic achievement. As many as 6 credits may be transferred from other schools.	30
Business Administration Major Area. Applies the decision-making and problem-solving lessons of the liberal arts in organizational environments. Up to 6 credits may be transferred.	30
Electives. Transferred in or selected by student in consultation with an advisor.	60
Two BS Degrees. Liberal arts and business administration. Replaces 30 credits of electives with second major.	0
Total	120
BS and MBA. MBA courses replace 30 undergraduate credits. Additional MBA credits.	6
Total	126

BACHELOR'S DEGREE IN LIBERAL ARTS OR BUSINESS ADMINISTRATION

A student may choose a single degree based upon a liberal arts foundation enriched by electives, as shown in figure 9.2.

TWO BACHELOR'S DEGREES

A student may choose two BS degrees, as shown in figure 9.3.

TRANSFER STUDENTS

The program also offers flexibility for transfer students, as shown in figure 9.4.

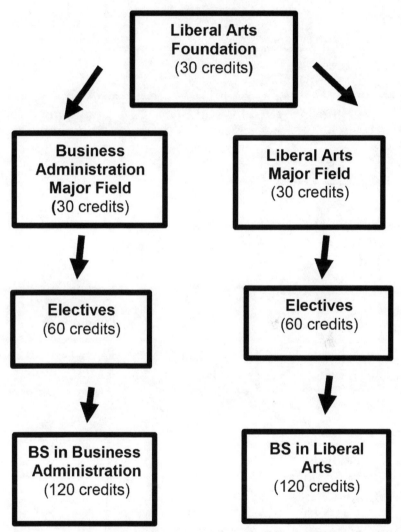

Figure 9.2. Pathway to a Liberal Arts or Business Administration Degree

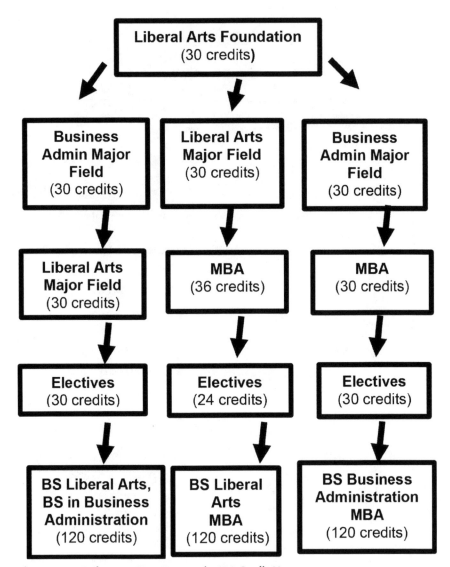

Figure 9.3. Pathway to Two Degrees in 120 Credit Hours

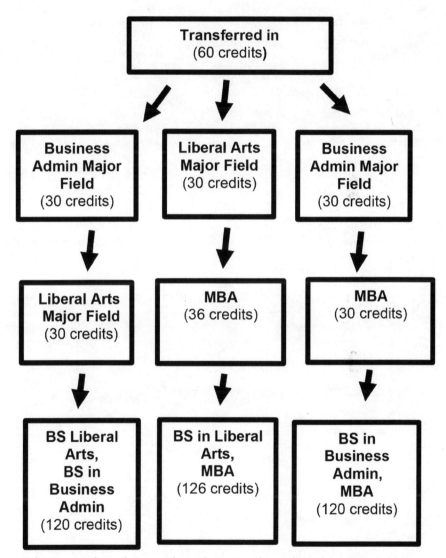

Figure 9.4.   Pathway for an Undergraduate Transfer Student with 60 Prior Credits

FLEXIBLE FORMATS AND GRADING FOR COURSES

For all of the courses, let's allow a structure that can accommodate three different formats. For a 3-credit class that would be scheduled traditionally to meet twice a week for seventy-five minutes for twelve weeks (twenty-four sessions), the formats would be the following:

- Blended (hybrid): Coursework is divided into attendance in person and a distance-learning component. Students attend half the previous number of class sessions in person (twelve sessions) and complete outside assignments to make up for the reduced in-person instruction.
- Remote: The same as hybrid, except the "in-person" sessions use Zoom or another conferencing technology.
- Online: Students take the class asynchronously, communicating electronically with the instructor.

In all formats, grading will be based on a midterm and final written exam/assignment covering material in a syllabus, textbook, other references or distributed materials, and asynchronous videos. Grading variations include the following:

- Hybrid or remote: An extra written submission required for each missed class or Zoom session
- Online: A third written submission required, comprising the submissions for individuals who missed hybrid or remote sessions

Figure 9.5 shows the variations in formatting and grading.

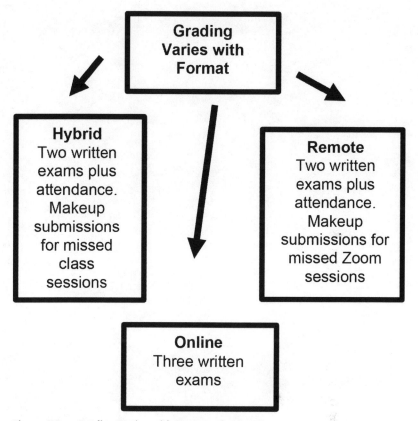

Figure 9.5.   Grading Varies with Format of a Course

CONCLUSION

Thus, we have a flexible program that retains the liberal arts foundation and offers options that meet the varying personal and professional situations of potential students. Now we just need to add a little more detail.

Chapter Ten

Authority, Responsibility, and Accountability in Business Continuity Planning: Who Should Be Responsible for What?

CURRICULUM DISCUSSIONS

With the academic structure in place and aligned with resources, the focus shifts as the institution digs down into curriculum design. Many choices exist. Differing points of view can be expected and should be respected. The process should be consistent with academic management overall. That structure involves responsibilities for the board of trustees, the president, deans, and professors.

BOARD OF TRUSTEES RESPONSIBILITIES

Regardless of a university's health, type, or status, business continuity planning needs trustee oversight. Figure 10.1 spells out the role of the board.

- Establish the organization's vision, mission, and purpose: Does the university need to rewrite its vision, mission, or values statements to enhance business continuity?
- Hire, monitor, and evaluate the chief executive: Does the institution have the right president to implement a continuity plan?
- Provide financial oversight: Does the plan contain a sustainable budget and adequate internal controls on incoming and outgoing funds?
- Ensure the adequacy of resources: Does the plan allocate money and other resources properly to achieve its goals?
- Approve the business continuity plan: Does the plan set the right objectives and steps to follow it? Is it likely to succeed?

• Ensure ethical behavior and legal compliance: Does the plan align with ethical principle and legal obligations?

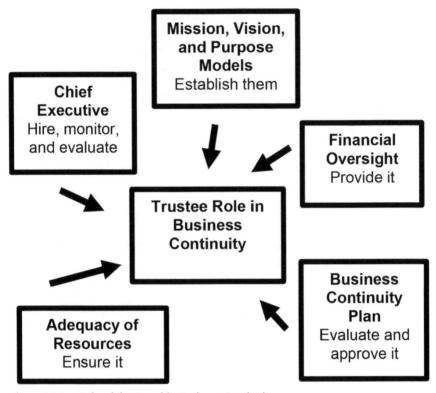

Figure 10.1.   Role of the Board in Business Continuity

RESPONSIBILITIES OF THE UNIVERSITY OFFICERS

The president, deans, other senior administrators, and faculty have roles to play in business continuity. The business contingency framework needs to be matched to the financial resources of the institution. Academic programs must comply with academic standards, resources, and capabilities to deliver the proper instructional content.

Returning now to the academic design of our credit programs of 120 to 126 hours, let's look at more details.

BS IN LIBERAL ARTS MAJOR

The liberal arts core can be designed in terms of traditional academic areas that match the degrees of existing professors. One approach to continuity planning is to create and require courses in specific liberal arts disciplines.

As an example, Nicholas Lemann, a Columbia University professor, proposes a liberal arts design that does not follow traditional academic areas of content. As figure 10.2 shows, it consists of eight courses that might be included in the liberal arts major.

INFORMATION ACQUISITION 101

Where do we go to separate beliefs, facts, assumptions, opinions, emotions, and bias? What makes up usable information? How do we distinguish whether academic, documentary, journalistic, governmental, and media information is true or false, reliable or questionable?

CAUSE AND EFFECT 101

How do we use the scientific method to find relationships? As an example: "Why do children in rural areas of India do poorly in school? Is it because they are not being fed properly at home?" What research could answer the question?

INTERPRETATION OF WRITTEN MEANING 101

How do we approach written content to identify and understand what it means? Students search for the obvious, the subtle, the hidden, and the missing. Start with a passage in the Constitution, the Bible, or a novel. What does it say? What is its meaning? What does it imply? What can we infer?

NUMERICAL LITERACY 101

What skills are needed to make sense out of numbers? What insights are not visible in raw data? What are the sources of numbers and what do they mean?

PERSONAL PERSPECTIVES 101

What do you believe about yourself and your world? Do others agree with you? Why is it so difficult to display tolerance, respect, and understanding when challenged by others?

VISUAL LANGUAGE 101

How do we develop and process information in the form of graphics instead of text or numbers? How do we use visual information to create positive responses?

THINKING IN TIME 101

How do we understand and apply knowledge to things that are happening? Students insert themselves into past situations. What would they have done? What should be done?

ARGUMENTATION 101

How do we take positions, draw conclusions, and explain our beliefs to others? What makes a compelling argument?

BUSINESS ADMINISTRATION MAJOR OUTCOMES

The business administration major could also be designed so its 30 credits are built around outcomes. Figure 10.3 identifies learning outcomes in several categories.

- Communications skills: Demonstrate written and oral skills in a business context.
- Management knowledge: Apply it in for-profit and nonprofit organizational settings.
- Problem solving: Collect data and use analytical tools to pursue strategic and operational goals.
- Develop business models: Identify and evaluate effective courses of action and ethical business practices.

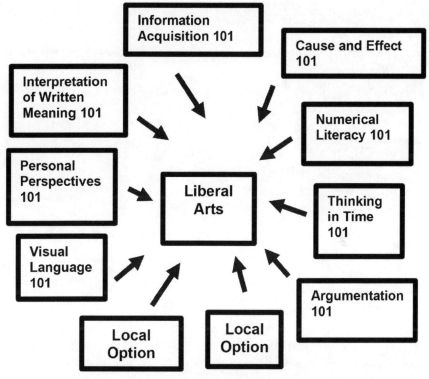

Figure 10.2.   Lemann's Approach to Liberal Arts Outcomes

- Risk management: Recognize both opportunities and risks in organizational decision making.

BUSINESS CONTINUITY PLAN FOR THE MBA

In a similar approach, business continuity planning applies to graduate degrees. The plan can match candidate backgrounds, needs, and goals to programs that offer value and flexibility. Figure 10.4 is an example in an MBA program of 36 total credits.

- MBA concentrations: Financial management or healthcare administration.
- Recruiting message: Our graduate business degrees provide breadth of knowledge from MBA courses and depth of knowledge from MS courses.
- Curriculum core courses: A candidate would choose 15 credits from a selection of 24 credits to fit with individual prior background and goals.
- Concentration: Three courses (9 credits) in finance or healthcare.

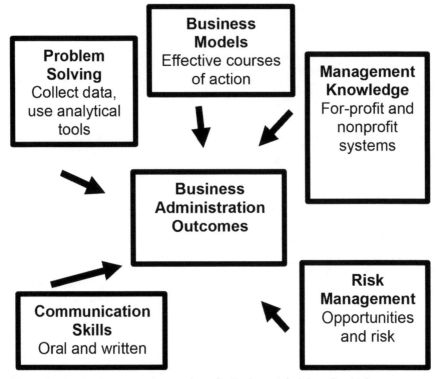

Figure 10.3.   An Outcomes Approach to the Business Administration Major

- Two concentrations: Three courses in the other concentration (9 credits)
- Electives: Three to 12 credits, depending upon the number of concentrations

MBA COURSE FORMATS

The programs would offer a combination of blended, remote, and distance learning to match the needs and goals of likely students.

MBA MARKETING EFFORT

The business continuity plan could recommend revised marketing efforts to promote graduate degrees. A specific attempt could use word-of-mouth messaging asking supporters and friendly communities to spread the word that flexible graduate business degrees have been designed for fast-track completion. Figure 10.5 shows targets for the marketing effort.

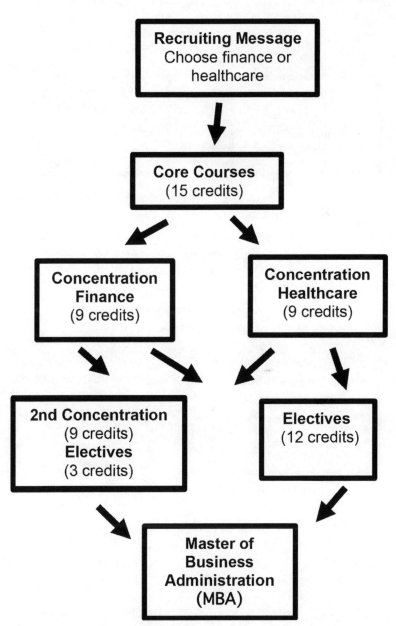

Figure 10.4. A 36-Credit MBA Design

- Current students
- Alumni
- Employers
- Other supporters

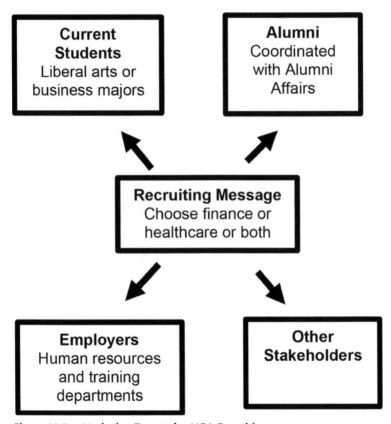

Figure 10.5. Marketing Targets for MBA Recruiting

CONCLUSION

Whatever the design and goals, a business continuity plan should involve the right individuals to make contributions to its various parts. As the authority, responsibility, and accountability are spread among the board, administrators, professors, students, and other stakeholders, the process should include roles for these interested parties.

Chapter Eleven

End of the Journey: What Would Happen If No One Listened to the Crisis in Higher Education?

FRAMEWORK OF RISK AND UNCERTAINTY

As we reach the end of our journey, I, like everyone else in higher education, am trapped in the post-COVID-19 higher education nightmare. It is tempting to blame many of today's college and university problems on the uncertainty wrought by the infectious respiratory virus. This would not be accurate.

Our story follows my earlier writings published in *Risk and Insurance* magazine. Three of the four articles, dated 2018 to 2020, were not about COVID-19. The titles tell us a serious problem existed.

- "Universities Face Dire Financial Risks during COVID-19. So Do Parents and College-Aged Students Who Make the Wrong Choices" (June 5, 2020)
- "20 Percent of Private Nonprofit Colleges Got a 'D' in Financial Health. How Quickly Can They Upgrade to a 'C'?" (April 14, 2020)
- "This Is Why Most Universities Get an 'F' in Risk Management" (February 1, 2019)
- "Will 600 Colleges Disappear in the Next 10 Years?" (August 8, 2018)

EVALUATING BUSINESS CONTINUITY EFFORTS

Now the story has been told and the challenge has been made to boards of trustees, college presidents, deans, and professors. Some questions should be addressed to them, including the following:

- Does your institution have a viable business model?
- Do your mission, vision, and values statements align with a viable business model?
- Are the trustees, administrators, and professors working together on strategies for the future?
- Do you have a business continuity plan?
- If yes, does it use an enterprise risk management approach to dealing with risk and uncertainty?
- Is it aligned with a viable business model?

As has been noted throughout the earlier pages, this book is focused largely on critical thinking and problem solving as it evolves from a liberal arts–based education. This brings a new series of questions, particularly for institutions built on a liberal arts foundation:

- Does your institution offer liberal arts courses in a sustainable value chain?
- Does your curriculum design respond to students' goals and needs?
- What do your students want?
- Does your business model and philosophy respond to the factors shape student choices of colleges and motivate them to attend your institution?

Another series of questions deals with the actual academic offerings of an institution:

- Do you have a modern curriculum containing and surrounding the liberal arts framework?
- Are you offering flexible formats for courses?
- Are you offering flexible structures for students to choose options that meet their goals and needs?
- Do your recruiting messages, admission requirements, graduation flexibility, course formats and schedules, and financial aid policies support and enrich your recruiting efforts?

Our remaining questions deal with authority, responsibility, and accountability in business continuity planning:

- Are the trustees performing their appropriate governance role?
- Are the administrators developing the right business continuity plans?
- Do professors, students, and other stakeholders concur with and support business continuity efforts?

A FINAL THOUGHT

For many colleges and universities, and particularly for private liberal arts institutions, the problems will not immediately go away. The need for business continuity is obvious across higher education, both from the perspective of the realities facing trustees, administrators, professors, students, parents, and others, and from any listing of financial and other dangers confronting us.

This brings to mind a quote that might give us some urgency: "More than any other time in history, higher education faces a crossroads. One path leads to despair and utter hopelessness. The other, to total extinction. Let us pray we have the wisdom to choose correctly."

I confess to a little dishonesty here. The quote is actually not about higher education. It led off a fictional "Speech to the Graduates" written by Woody Allen for the *New York Times* in 1979. It refers to mankind and was made in a comedic context. Still, it reminds us that we need to choose the right path when we come to any juncture in the road. We are at that point dealing with the future of many of today's colleges and universities.

On this note, we have reached the end of our journey.

Index

About the Author

John "Jack" Hampton is professor of business at St. Peter's University in New Jersey and a core faculty member at the International School of Management (Paris). He was executive director of the Risk and Insurance Management Society (RIMS), dean of the schools of business at Seton Hall and Central Connecticut State universities, and provost of the College of Insurance and SUNY Maritime College. He holds master's and doctoral degrees in business and finance from George Washington University.

AWARDS

Risk Innovator of 2008, *Risk and Insurance* magazine
2011 Innovation Award, *Business Insurance* magazine
Handbook of Financial Risk Management, Outstanding Business Reference
    Book of 2012, American Library Association
2018 Risk All-Star Award, *Risk and Insurance* magazine

RISK MANAGEMENT IN HIGHER EDUCATION

Hampton is author of a Rowman & Littlefield series on risk management in higher education. Previous publications include the following:

Culture, Intricacies, and Obsessions in Academia: Why Colleges and Universities Are Struggling to Deliver the Goods (2017)
The Professoriate Today: Languishing in Dante's Purgatory (2017)

Liberal Arts in the Doldrums: Rethink, Revise, and Revitalize to Reverse the Trend (2017)

The Malaise of Academic Scholarship: Why It Starts with the Doctoral Dissertation as a Baptism of Fire (2017)

EARLIER RISK MANAGEMENT PUBLICATIONS

Prior to concentrating on higher education, he published in the areas of finance and risk management. Hampton's books by the American Management Association are as follows:

Essentials of Risk Management and Insurance
Financial Management of Insurance Companies
AMA Management Handbook, 3rd edition (general editor)
Enterprise Risk Management (two editions)
AMA Handbook of Financial Risk Management

His books by other publishers include the following:

Evaluating Shipping Transactions
Economics of Ocean Transportation
Financial Decision Making (four editions)
Handbook for Financial Decision Makers
Modern Financial Theory
Corporate Finance Using an Electronic Spreadsheet
Working Capital Management